T0369080

LIFE
WITHOUT
DIABETES—
FACT OR FICTION?

LIFE WITHOUT DIABETES—
FACT OR FICTION?

A TOTAL Body Makeover
from the INSIDE OUT

MICHELLE D' ANGEL

iUniverse, Inc.
New York   Bloomington

iUniverse books may be ordered through booksellers or by contacting:

iUniverse
1663 Liberty Drive
Bloomington, IN 47403
www.iuniverse.com
1-800-Authors (1-800-288-4677)

ISBN: 978-1-4401-5316-7 (sc)
ISBN: 978-1-4401-5314-3 (dj)
ISBN: 978-1-4401-5315-0 (ebook)

Printed in the United States of America

iUniverse rev. date: 11/18/2009

*I like to dedicate this book to all of you that have been struggling
with yo-yo dieting, and trying to control your diabetic condition.*

I would recommend this book for anyone who has diabetes. It is very informative and provides sensible regimens for nutrition and exercise. This" Total Body Makeover" will improve the quality of life for people with diabetes.

Michael P. Mortire M.D.

Contents

Acknowledgments

My deepest thanks to the hard working and dedicated people who have supported, encouraged, and inspired me.

Many thanks goes out to my husband for trusting me and accepting to be my guinea pig, trying different foods and recipes, in this endeavor to a life free from medication and diabetes. Also, it is because of him I start writing this book.

Thanks to my daughter, whose belief in the importance of this book and my ability to write it, kept me going every step of the way.

To my parents and my mother in low, which I wish they will still be around to see this book published—you will be so proud!

Thanks goes out to Michael Epps, for his help in the process of editing this book.

Thanks to all the friends and parents for trying my recipes. Their feedback helped me to select the best recipes for this book.

Introduction

There are reasons for our sadness and happiness. Our lives are like a fast ride on a carousel, with many ups, downs, and sudden stops. We begin this ride as early as child as we rebel against the rules set forth by our families. We resign the friends that don't tell us what we want to hear, get our hearts broken or break someone else's heart, but we seem to move on. We have some scars, but we shake them off, the same way a dog shakes the water out of his fur. That is life!

But what happens when we become adults? Innocence can no longer protect us, as we are expected to know and fix it all. But, what if we haven't been taught properly? What if everything that we've learned up to this point has failed? What do we do? I say you get informed, and this is just the book to do that.

Though recommended, it is not necessary to read the entire book. Like the Yellow Pages you may have direct access according to your needs. This book contains everything you need to know in helping to progress from a life of diabetes to a life of wholeness. It won't overwhelm you with statistics; it is the actual account of an ordinary person living with Type 2 diabetes.

You will hear of the everyday struggles and challenges which were faced. You will also hear of the successful and unsuccessful attempts made to overcome this illness. But, in the end the greatest part of this story to be told is the victory of managing and even overcoming Type 2 Diabetes.

Chapter One

HOW IT ALL BEGAN

Face to Face With Destiny

I will always remember how I met my husband. We were in our home land of Romania at a business dinner. This dinner was being held at the very luxurious Romanian hotel known as the Intercontinental. It was out of curiosity that I decided to attend this meeting to learn more about new forms of energy, a subject that intrigued me as an economist. If I remember correctly, there were close to two hundred people at this meeting, representing various countries, cultures, and cuisine. The meal was scrumptious! The menu was graced by rich and tasty appetizers, and five main courses. Lights and formal dressings decorated the ballroom. *What more could I wish for?*

As I savored the sautéed jumbo shrimp and snow crab legs, some of my favorite foods, little did I know that my future husband was sitting right in front of me. He was tall, with dark hair, and bright eyes that were staring right at me. At that moment my whole life was spinning like a carousel.

Unlike myself, I noticed he was eating only a plain salad. I thought to myself, as my eyes surveyed the table, a "plain salad?" I guess because of my expression, is why he simply looked at me and smiled.

Later that night, he asked me to dance, and while were dancing, I found out why he was eating only a salad—he had diabetes. Diabetes was no surprise to me, because my father had diabetes, so I wasn't afraid of the subject. In fact, I felt pretty knowledgeable when it came to diabetes, but I would soon find, that I still had a lot to learn.

Needless to say, that was the beginning of our life together, because four months later, he and I were married. And, so began our journey in attempting to manage and live with Type 2 diabetes.

Life with Diabetes

When I first met my husband, he didn't display the "typical" signs of Type 2 diabetes (we shall discuss these in later chapters). To begin with, though he had a bit of a belly that seemed somewhat complimentary to the emergent gray hair on the side of his head, which is typical of a 39 year old man, he was still tall and *lean*.

As a couple, we were physically active; both of us were former gymnasts, and we now own and coach a gymnastic club. We made sure that we ate a healthy, and balanced home-cooked meals. We did everything to maintain a healthy lifestyle. But, despite our attempt, my husband's diabetes worsened. As a result, like most people I began to seriously wonder, "What could be the problem?" This particular question would be the motivation to prompt my future research.

My husband took on a regular basis Glyburide to help the release of his body's natural insulin, and Metformin to restore his body's response to insulin. However, the medications seemed to no longer work. He often even increased his dosage, but his blood sugar level still increased. "*What were we not doing?*" We had found a doctor who was knowledgeable, patient, and wiling to listen and discuss our problems. We made sure we maintained regular visits with him for check-ups and blood work. We followed our doctor's advice and his emphases on eating healthy and exercising, which was pretty much what we were already doing, but it was to no avail.

With the constant rising of his blood sugar level reaching 300-400, my husband's body underwent significant changes. He developed a big appetite, and gained a lot of weight around his midsection. He went through an emotional state, where he experienced mood swings, and became very nervous and impatient. He experienced head sweats, leg cramps, fatigue, and low endurance. And, to make things worse, his cholesterol, blood pressure, and triglycerides levels continued escalating.

At that point, we turned to specialists and nutritionists. We followed their diets and every other diet on the market at that time, but still nothing. My husband's blood sugar level simply would not go down, despite already being at a maximum dosage of medication. And, though, he was dealing with Type 2 diabetes, and not Type 1, our doctor tried insulin as a last resort. The insulin caused his blood sugar level to skyrocket as high as 500. Now, we had tried everything we could think of, but nothing worked.

Our lives were dramatically affected by this. It felt as if my life, and the man I had married and loved, were changed forever. We had no answers, and we were both suffering. It was as if I had awakened one morning in a different place and time. Was this the beginning of the END?

We Panicked!

My husband's condition didn't improve at all. He began to have trouble with his breathing, and developed chest pains. His feet became swollen, red, and painful. At some point, our doctor recommended a stress test, because he was concerned about his heart. My husband went to take the stress test, but couldn't perform it. The stress test consists of having to walk on a treadmill at various speeds and levels, while being monitored by a heart monitor. My husband, unfortunately, couldn't seem to walk long enough due to his breathing, to complete the test. So, the cardiologist then suggested that an angiogram be done.

The cardiologist suspected that there might be a high percentage of blockages in his arteries. This possibility was frightening. I went and I did my homework to learn more about what an angiogram entailed, and from that research I became afraid of the risks that were involved. This made me hesitant, so I went and talked with the cardiologist. He convinced me that the angiogram had to be done, and that the risk of not doing it, was greater than the risk of doing it.

While preparing for the procedure at the hospital, the doctor presented me with several papers to sign, including release and permission forms requesting authorization for "open heart surgery!" For a moment, I couldn't breathe. I attempted to try and console myself, by kindly reminding the doctor of his early encouragement regarding my husband's safety, and the necessity of this angiogram. I tried to somehow quizzically assure myself that it would not, in fact, be dangerous. He pointed out that he expected a significant amount of blockage in his arteries up to 90%, due to the way my husband reacted to the stress test. I was really scared! What would this mean?

As I stood there, I began thinking to myself, "Anything could possibly happen at this point, and we have no other family here besides our children." I suddenly realized how much I missed having my extended family nearby. I felt so all alone. I didn't know to whom or where to turn for comfort.

The time I spent waiting on my husband to return from that angiogram, felt more like an eternity than the five hours that had past. Finally, they brought him back, and the doctor came to talk to us wearing a big smile on his face. His smile was comforting, but his news was even better. He said that there was only a 30% blockage in one of my husband's arteries. He assured us that the diagnosis could be managed with proper medication and diet. I was thrilled!

The Beginning of the End

What is Diabetes?

I was confused for a while as to what we were actually dealing with. My biggest question was, "What's really the problem?" Though we tried everything, we still couldn't control the sugar level, blood pressure, or cholesterol. And, to make matters worse, my husband began developing heart problems, and that was frightening! I was now both scared and confused.

It was hard to watch his suffering, and not know what to do to help him. I could see that he was really feeling bad. His energy was gone, and this was causing him to tire very easy. His legs were often hurting, though he tried to hide it. But, above all, I could see that the outward manifestations of what he was dealing with, was nothing in comparison to what he was dealing with on the inside. It seemed as if daily he was becoming more and more frustrated. He was sad, and no longer had a desire for anything. It was as though he was dying inside.

I, on the other hand, still had no answers, or understanding as to what was going on. That's when I realized that in fact, knew very little about diabetes, especially Type 2 diabetes. I now had a lot of questions, and only a few answers. For starters:

- Who are the people that get diabetes?
- What is the cause of diabetes?
- Are there any cures for diabetes?
- Is there any difference between Type 2 diabetes, insulin resistance, and Syndrome X?

All the information that I had about diabetes was confusing. Since we tried so many avenues before, and nothing worked, I knew that if I wanted to help my husband, I had to find answers to my questions. It then occurred to me that this entire time, we had been trying to address *his condition* of diabetes, and not the *cause*. I quickly realized that we needed to change our approach. Instead, of addressing to the problem, we needed to get to *the root* of the problem. That was the beginning of my studies on diabetes.

I went to the library and bookstores. I bought all the books I could find on diabetes and nutrition. I was really surprised at how many books I found on the subject. I had no idea that there was so much information out there. For some, this might have frightened them with so much medical information, but being that I grew up in a family of doctors, I was already familiar with a lot of medical terminologies and definitions. Besides, learning how to research to find specific information is one of the first things you learn in college.

After about 6 months of continuous study and research, I had finally seen the light. I now knew what Type 2 diabetes was, and its operation in the body. From there I continued on with my studies, reading up on various treatments pertaining to Type 2 diabetes, and the possibilities of being reversed. From my study, I found out alarming information about this disease.

Facts about Diabetes

According to the Center of Disease Control and Prevention (CDC, 2007):

- 24 million people which represent 8% of population currently have diabetes in the United States, and this number is steady on the rise.
- 57 million people are estimated to have prediabetes.
- Diabetes is the 7th leading cause of death in the United States.
- It is estimated that more than 95% of people diagnosed with diabetes, have Type 2 diabetes.
- Diabetics are more likely to develop blindness, kidney problems, nerve disease, limb amputation, heart problems, and cerebral hemorrhaging.

————— Chapter Two —————

KNOWLEDGE IS THE KEY TO SUCCESS

Life is a continuous process of learning and growth. Whether that learning is gained from previous life lessons and mistakes, or through the intentional acquiring of knowledge, we gain what is needed to make the necessary adjustments in life. This approach is both true in relationships, careers, and even our health and body. When it comes to the betterment of life—*knowledge is the key.*

Knowledge gives us the power to make informed decisions. With the abundance of information available through the media, we are surely not without help. You can find information on everything, from weight loss and improved sleep quality, to how to better your sex life. And even when it comes to diabetes, there is an abundance of information as well.

However, many of the advertisements claim to be "sure fire" or "scientifically proven," but my question is, *"Proven for whom?"* When studies claim diabetics are permitted to have moderate sugar servings, *"What is moderation?"* Is moderate for me, the same as moderate for you? Though much of the advice is good, it's sometimes good only for a handful of people, often only the ones whom the products have been "clinically" tested on.

As everyday people, it is part of our nature to want to eagerly try that which sounds like good and practical information. Unfortunately, we fail to see the *fine print* stating the possible consequences and *side effects* of many of the publicized products.

We also fail to *read thoroughly* the *disclaimers* which are presented, to see if these products are detrimental to our condition—condition such as diabetes, kidney and heart complications. Many of these products exclude a lot of us, especially those of us who are getting older and dealing with some of these problems. Becoming educated to the facts, will save you time and money, but above all, it will empower you to make informed decisions.

Now days, due to the unseen side effects that tend to emerge from many medications, there have been an ongoing recall of many of them. Many of these medications have shown true that while they do attempt to successfully resolve the main conditions we face, they are often damaging to other areas of the body. And, while this might be profitable for the lawyers out there, for the people who have already exhausted time and money in a desperate quest for health, this delays the intended outcome, and adds stress to the load. All of us must decide to either take the publicized "*quick fix*" with all its risk, or address the root of the problem in a safe and healthy way.

Learning about our body and its functions, will help minimize the confusion often times found through being uninformed. Understanding bridges the confusion gap of language and terminologies, often found between doctors and patients. Being informed becomes as much of an important part of recovery, as the medication we take.

If you are one of the people who rely on the offered information of others as a soother to the mind, you might want to think again. Often times the information given to us by advertisements or doctors is partial and foreign to our understanding. I remember back when my husband first started to deal with all of this, the residential doctor at the hospital, came to me, and said that my husband had pneumonia, and that his cholesterol was also high. And, then when I asked him what the reading was, with a slight arrogance in his voice, he asked me if I was familiar with the cholesterol readings, I said "Yes." He then said, in a plain but blunt way, "Well, your husband's cholesterol is 225," then turned and went into the examining room. I was left standing there with a feeling of anger and incompleteness.

Finally, after nearly five hours of sitting in that busy emergency room waiting area, with little or no feedback, my husband was admitted to his room. This would have been a good thing, except for the unfortunate reality of having to wait even longer to have our questions answered by the doctor. I guess due to the work load and many cases that the doctors have to deal with, is why when he finally arrived, his attitude seemed somewhat routine and even insulting in ways. During that time, I didn't have the resources and understanding as I do now. So, you can imagine being well informed by him was the key to our peace. But, in my opinion, his care and consideration for his patient appeared somewhat lacking.

This was just a demonstration to show that whether you have a good doctor or the occasional bad one, being *personally* informed is power. Knowing is critical in all situations, especially when dealing with doctors and their many terminologies. Or, perhaps knowing simply helps you to be in better control of your body and its functions. As, the old adage goes, "*When you know better, you can do better.*"

Knowing is Power

There is no one treatment that seems to fit us all, just as there is no one food pyramid that's beneficial to everyone. Each and every one of us are genetically, metabolically, physically, and physiologically different. Learning this is beneficial in helping us choose foods that are favorable for our condition.

In the beginning, after only a very short time, my husband and me, came against many controversial recommendations made by specialists in the field, which left us with the task of trying to know which one to follow. We tried many of the diets on the market, switching from high protein diets to high carbohydrates diets, and eventually to low-fat diets. With all the diets and books out there written by specialists, you could best believe there were going to be contradictions of opinions. For example, it was initially said that eggs were not good for you, but when later reviewed, specialists came back and stated that eggs in fact were beneficial to your diet. As a result of the inconsistencies of their statements, you can imagine this brought on frustration.

When it comes to nutrition this is a relatively new field, with many still unanswered questions. Questions like, "*Why only certain people in the obese weight class get diabetes?*" "*Why some people more then others are prone to certain diseases?*" Even with a wealth of accessible information, there are many things still unresolved.

The bottom line is we're all different, and until we stop blaming genetics, ancestry or simply life in general, and get to know ourselves and what is good for us, there will always remain health issues. It is imperative that we begin to know what foods and vitamins are right for us, what exercises are right for us, and even what relationship is right for us. These are all key factors towards a healthy life.

At some point, the same way we have given unconditional love to our spouse, children, and all the other things we treasure, we must learn to equally give that same commitment toward the wholeness of our body.

The Things We Need to Know

1. What is Type 2 Diabetes?

Type 2 diabetes is a metabolic condition. It is caused by our genes, lack of physical activity, by the foods we eat, and how we process those foods. With Type 2 diabetes, there is no defect in insulin production. This simply means that the pancreas is fully functional, often times making anywhere from enough insulin to more then enough. Type 2 diabetes is a result of our body's inability to effectively use the insulin. According to some doctors, Type 2 diabetes could have a low insulin production. Insulin is a hormone secreted by the pancreas in response to rising blood sugar levels during the digestion of food.

All the carbohydrates that we eat are at some point broken down into glucose. Proteins and fats can also be used to make glucose. Glucose is our body's primary fuel. Insulin is essential for glucose circulating in the bloodstream to enter the cells, where it supplies the energy to run the functions of the body. If the action of insulin is blocked, glucose cannot be removed from the blood stream. This in turn, causes the glucose level to rise, and cells to starve, ultimately resulting in a diabetic condition.

Type 2 diabetes is characterized by poor insulin sensitivity. This means that cells do not respond to insulin signals, therefore they do not take up nutrients from the blood stream as well as they should.

Blood sugar level is the common name used, to represent the concentration, or level of glucose in the bloodstream. If glucose cannot enter the cells, it remains in the bloodstream, thereby resulting in high sugar level readings.

Characteristics of Type 2 Diabetes:

- • Central obesity
- • High cholesterol
- • High blood pressure
- • High triglycerides
- • High ratio of bad to good cholesterol

- ❖ A closer look at Appendix 1 will show you the results

of my husband's blood work, which bore all of these particular characteristics.

The Following are Believed to Cause Insulin Insensitivity

- Poor diet
- Obesity or high proportion of fat in body tissues
- Inactivity/Sedentary lifestyle
- Deficiencies of certain vitamins and minerals

2. Why is Diabetes Dangerous?

Type 2 diabetes can be referred to as a multifaceted condition. The *frightening part* about this disease *is not the general feeling or symptoms* such as: chronic fatigue, poor digestion, aching joints, tender muscles, depression, food cravings, chest discomfort, shortness of breath, *but the long-term complications* resulting from uncontrolled blood sugar such as: blindness or vision impairment, irreversible nerve damage, kidney failure, heart disease, and early death. From what I have read, there is no medication in the world that can stop the diabetes progression, but only to some degree slow it down. Having Type 2 diabetes over time *ultimately alters the quality of life.*

3. Medication is Not the Answer

In the beginning, prior to being "informed," I actually believed the medication my husband was taking was enough. I figured we could eat out and still indulge in some of the richer foods as long as he took his medication. Back then, I was almost in a naive state, believing in the ability of medicine to "magically" solve the problem, and that going to the doctor and following the prescribed regimen would be sufficient. Wow, was I wrong!

Through my research, I found out that all doctors agree that drugs are not safe. All drugs taken over a long period of time have side effects, which affect the heart, kidney or liver, and even the immune system. This would have been great information to know back then.

My dad recently died from a heart attack. He also had Type 2 diabetes which, at that time I never understood why he acquired it. Looking back over my father's lifestyle, he never ate sweets, and he always had his coffee or tea unsweetened. Back then, our living was healthier, we were lucky not to have fast food places in Romania, so it was the norm to eat good home-cooked meals. Due to low industrialized agriculture during that time, most of our food was naturally grown. He also adhered to his doctor's guidelines about his diet: eliminating fats and fried foods, and eating lots of vegetables, fruits, salads, and whole grain bread.

A few years before he died, he came to visit us over the holidays. When he came, I notice he had a chart of medications, in which he had to take daily. Besides the medication for diabetes, he had one medication for the heart, another for the liver, and so on. Looking at his medical records, and reading the medication' prospects, I was able to see that his kidney problem was related to diabetes, but was aggravated by one of the medication that he took. In fact, most of the medications set off an entire chain of events that were irreversible, which I believe led up to his heart attack.

4. Proper Diet a Must for Diabetics

As mentioned, according to doctors, Type 2 diabetes is a metabolic condition characterized by poor insulin sensitivity. Simply put, it's the body inability to properly process the food we eat.

From the time of learning that medications are more harmful than helpful, I've been left with one conclusion: nutrition should be the one controllable variable that should be addressed. In other words, we *first* have to obtain and maintain an adequate diet, and let medication become secondary.

Increasing insulin sensitivity

If you look at the factors that lead to insulin insensitivity, you will see that they are rather interrelated. Poor dieting, and inactivity leads to obesity, and obesity precludes inactivity. In other words, the bigger or heavier you are, the harder it is to exercise.

Below is an outlined plan devise for my husband, based on the knowledge I acquired:

- Losing weight is essential.
- Find a diet that works from the sugar level point of view, containing foods that are appealing, and that can be maintain for life.
- Exercise is a big "must."

- Take time to find the right vitamins and mineral supplements for his body.

Obesity

One thing that doesn't cease to surprise me is the amount of overweight children that attend our gymnastics facility each day. Parents bring their children to gymnastics hoping they will get exercise and lose weight. Unfortunately, I noticed these same parents arriving to pick their kids up carrying fast food.

Through the many years of gymnastics, and having countless kids on competitive levels, we have seen kids of all body types, from the leanest to the heaviest. But for many parents, this was surprising because they thought gymnastics was for smaller leaner kids. As I've always told them, the body size really doesn't matter, as much as the development of muscles to carry that body.

Obesity is considered the major cause of Type 2 diabetes. But when it comes to dealing with obesity and losing weight, I try to avoid giving direct advice. Instead I share common-sense suggestions such as eating less sugar, bread, pasta, and fat. Remember, simple changes bring sure results, and it's up to each one of us to make the decision to maintain a healthy lifestyle.

Finding the right diet

Selecting the appropriate diet can be difficult, with so many diets on the market. I can recall my husband and me trying everything from high-carbohydrate diets to diets high in protein, but none of these seemed to work. I then decided that a balanced diet would be the right answer, but the problem was how to find the right balance. I had seen all the popular diets endorsed by the doctors and nutritionists, and knew they were tested by large groups of people, but I didn't have the time or the paid volunteers. So, I decide to use my husband as the guinea pig. To me, this seemed like the only option.

First, I had to find out why all the other diets failed to work for him. So I started on what I like to call a "food elimination diet." He was allowed to try different foods, and based on his sugar level response, this would determine whether or not we kept or eliminated those particular foods. We kept foods that resulted in little or no sugar increase, and eliminated foods that resulted in a greater increase of the blood sugar level. This food elimination diet helped me to create our own food pyramid, which has shown to be beneficial.

Another component of the plan was to find the right vitamins and mineral supplement. Normally, when I go to the store, I am too busy to really read and examine *everything*. But, at some point I decided it was time for me to survey the store. While at the health food store, I found out the benefits of many items. On the vitamin shelf, I found a lot of *cleansers* for the body, liver, kidneys. This gave me an idea. First, my husband's body needed cleansing to eliminate toxins, and after that, we could start fresh with a balanced diet. The diet would be comprised of balanced amounts of lean proteins, carbohydrates provided mostly by vegetables, and the essential fats needed for proper physiological functions. The percentage of each group in the diet would be determined by how his body processed and responded to the specific foods.

Now, through being able to make informed decisions, I was starting to feel real good. The ball was finally starting to roll!

──────── Chapter Three ────────

NUTRITION AND NUTRIENTS

In a 1962 Medical School Conference on nutrition, nutrition was defined as a major concern having "certain social, economical, cultural and psychological implications on food and eating."(Fleck, 1981) Food is a basic necessity of life, and it is important for everyone to become well-informed about the role nutrition plays in everyday living. Nutrients are defined by specialists as substances that are necessary for the functioning of living organisms (Fleck, Introduction to Nutrition, 1981).

There are five major groups of nutrients: carbohydrates, proteins, fats, vitamins, and minerals. The foods we eat serve as our sole source of nutrients for the body. We have all heard the old adage, "you are what you eat," so knowing the kind and amount of nutrients in our diet is very important. Each nutrient plays a specific role, and research has established a recommended daily amount of each. Learning about nutrients in food is both interesting and important in knowing their role and function. Knowing the nutritional value of foods is the only way we can make and keep a healthy diet. For example, apples and table sugar are both examples of simple carbohydrates, but apples contain nutrients like pectin, which is a type of fiber that aids in lowering cholesterol.

At times, the task of having to learn such terms and definitions can become boring and tedious, but remember this: *the benefits are well worth the time and effort.*

A. Carbohydrates

As of lately, we're beginning to hear this word more and more. We hear the terms good carbs, and bad carbs, diets rich in carbs and diets low in carbs, but the one thing we hear very little about is what carbohydrates actually are? *What are the merits of carbohydrates, and their influence on our body? Which carbohydrates should we choose?*

In order to make the right choices, we must be informed! It is important to know why we should make any changes that could affect our lifestyle, before we actually make these changes. Knowing what carbohydrates are, how they are processed, and how they affect our body is very important to everybody, *especially diabetics.* Knowing "why" a bagel is bad for you, instead of simply hearing that it's bad, empowers you to make better food choices. While it may not sound exciting, it is important to understand carbohydrates, and the role they play in elevating the sugar level (blood glucose). In addition, it further helps to understand why exercise is so important in avoiding obesity.

Along with protein and fat, carbohydrates are one of the three groups of macronutrients that make up the human diet. All foods except fat contain carbohydrates. Some foods contain larger amounts than others. All carbohydrates contain sugar. Our body extracts sugar from carbohydrates, and transforms that sugar into glucose, which is either burned or stored as body fat. When sugars are absorbed too quickly into the bloodstream, this can cause problems for the diabetic.

The speed of digestion is determined by the chemical nature of carbohydrates. Carbohydrates consist of carbon, hydrogen and oxygen, which are in the same proportions as in water: two hydrogen molecules to one oxygen molecule. In terms of chemical structure, carbohydrates can be classified into three major groups:

1. Monosaccharides which are simple sugars, includes glucose, fructose, and galactose. Glucose also known as grape sugar, dextrose and corn sugar, is found in fruits, plant juice, milk and milk products. Fructose is found in fruits, vegetables, honey and cane sugar. Galactose is found in milk and milk products. The three monosaccharides are the end products of all digestible forms of carbohydrates.

2. Disaccharides yield two simple sugars upon the breakdown. They are sucrose, lactose and maltose. Sucrose, which is most widely distributed in foods, is composed of one molecule of glucose and one molecule of fructose. In its pure form it is found in table sugar, whether derived from sugar cane or sugar beets. Sucrose could also be found in fruits and plant juices, mixed with glucose and fructose. Lactose consists of equal parts of glucose and galactose, and is found in various amounts, in the milk of all mammal species. Maltose is composed of two molecules of glucose, and is a result of starch breakdown. During the germination or sprouting of cereal, a specific enzyme acts upon the starch and reduces it to maltose. Disaccharides are crystalline, sweet, and easily digested.

3. Polysaccharides yield more than two simple sugars upon the breakdown or digestion. The principal ones are starch, dextrin, glycogen, and cellulose. Starch is found in cereal grains, roots, bulbs, and tubers. Most plants store their food supply in the form of starch. As ripening takes place, the starch changes into glucose which gives sweet taste to ripe fruits. Dextrin is the intermediate product between starch and sugar. When bread is toasted, some of the starches become dextrin, generating a slightly sweet taste. Glycogen, frequently called animal starch, is the form of which animals and man store carbohydrates. Glycogen is stored in the human liver and small amounts are present in every body cell.

Another polysaccharide is fiber, and the major concern for humans is dietary fiber. The possible constituents of dietary fiber includes cellulose, which is found in small amounts in the wall of most plants, and pectin which is found in small amounts in the cell wall and in the rind of certain fruits such as oranges and apples. Another constituent is hemicelluloses, also found in cell wall, and has water-holding capacity.

Plants store sugar in a form of starch, whereas animal and humans can only store a limited amount of sugar as glycogen, in both the liver and the skeletal muscles. Starch and glycogen, unlike fiber, can be used by the body for the production of energy.

Carbohydrates are more easily converted into glucose than protein and fat. This is especially true for simple carbohydrates because their molecular structure breaks down faster. This ultimately raises the glucose level in the bloodstream quite rapid.

Simple carbohydrates (monosaccharides and disaccharides) and complex carbohydrates (polysaccharides) are broken down through digestion into simple sugars before being absorbed. They are absorbed by the small intestine, and travel to the liver where they are converted into glucose. Glucose is then either stored in the liver as glycogen or released into the bloodstream. Blood glucose levels are maintained primarily through the glycogen that is stored in the liver.

When the blood glucose is low, or during prolonged exercise when skeletal muscles are using it as fuel, glycogen from the liver is broken down into glucose by a process called "glycogenolysis." This process is facilitated by a hormone called glucagons which is released by the pancreas. The end result is the maintenance or increase of the blood glucose level. When blood glucose is high, glucose is taken up by the tissues with the help of a hormone called insulin, which is also released by the pancreas. When taken up by the liver, glucose can either be used for metabolism, or it can be converted and stored as glycogen. Glucose taken up by the skeletal muscles that's not used for metabolic purposes can be stored as muscular glycogen. If both the liver and the muscle glycogen stores are filled, excess glucose can be converted by the fat (adipose) cell to fat and stored as energy.

Carbohydrates are an indispensable source of energy since certain tissues require and use carbohydrates for fuel under all physiological conditions, especially the heart muscle. In addition to being a source of energy in the liver, carbohydrates have a protective and detoxifying action. Carbohydrates also have a regulating influence on protein and fat metabolism.

While the importance of carbohydrates from a health standpoint should not be minimized, knowing how much, and which ones we should have in our daily diet is imperative. The *Knowing Your Foods* chapter will help you to not only know your foods, but also help you to make your own selection in regards to the quantity and quality of carbohydrates in your diet.

Carbohydrates: *"Good or Bad?"*

During the process of studying and trying out different foods, and their affects on my husband's sugar level, I found that starchy carbohydrates such as bread, pasta, potatoes, and rice, raised his sugar level significantly. While on the other hand, those that were comprised of certain vegetables and fruits had little to no affect on his sugar level. I also learned that for diabetics, the quantity and the type of carbohydrates are very significant. This was later reflected in my husband's diet, and his ability to process starchy carbohydrates better when they were given in small amounts.

I personally consider simple carbohydrates and sugars to be addictive. The more we have them, the more we tend to want them. Sweets and chocolates gives us an energy rush for an hour or so, but when the effects wear off, we tend to need another piece to get that energy level back up. Complex carbohydrates from vegetables and fruits, gives us energy in smaller doses, but for longer periods of time, due to their slow absorption.

I remember growing up eating bread with almost every meal, and at the end of every meal it was also typical for me to have dessert. I kept these eating habits until recently. Though I was not a diabetic, I saw the necessity for change, due to an increased weight gain, which was a sure sign of my body no longer being able to properly process them.

It is sometimes difficult to imagine meals without such things as bread, pasta, rice, butter, bagels, sweets or potato chips, especially if we've become accustomed to eating them. Sometimes, the loss of certain foods tends to bring on a sense of loss or incompleteness when it comes to our meals.

If we could reprogram our way of thinking as easily as a computer, life would truly be easier. But unfortunately, we can't. It takes setting a clear goal, having a strong will, and doing everything in our power to achieve a healthy diet. We have to erase all preconceptions about foods that we haven't tried, and be open-minded to try and accept new foods in order to succeed.

B. Fiber

As of lately, we have all heard the hype about including fiber in our diets. Doctors and many television commercials advise us to increase our fiber intake. Apparently, fiber plays a role in preventing colon cancer, controlling cholesterol, and managing weight. Fiber is also essential in controlling glucose in diabetics. It holds nutrients in the intestinal tract longer, thereby slowing down the process of digestion. As a result, sugars are released into the bloodstream more gradually.

Digestion is the action of the stomach, in which foods are broken down to its components. Anything that speeds the process, by which the body digests carbohydrates can be a bad thing. The faster the sugars and starches (which are chains of sugars) are processed and absorbed into the bloodstream, the more weight we gain. Slower digestion of carbohydrates, results in less insulin being produced by the pancreas, which in turn reduces the ups and downs of the blood sugar level. Like fiber, fat, proteins, and acidic foods (e.g., lemon juice and vinegar) slow down digestion. As a result, this keeps us feeling fuller longer, which results in a smaller portion being eaten on our next meal.

But, what is fiber anyway? Dietary fiber is a complex carbohydrate. It is the part of a plant food that cannot be digested and absorbed in the bloodstream. There are two types of fiber: soluble and insoluble.

Soluble fiber dissolves and thickens in water to form a gel. A good source of soluble fiber includes dried beans, legumes, oatmeal, oat bran, barley, and citrus fruits. Research shows that this type of fiber may help lower blood cholesterol.

Insoluble fibers include the woody or structural part of plants such as fruit and vegetable skin, wheat bran, and whole wheat cereal. Insoluble fiber tends to speed the passage of material through the digestive tract, which also helps to prevent the risk of colon cancer. Eating foods with high fiber content will reduce the net carbohydrate intake. I will explain what I mean.

Let just say you are buying bread that has a total carbohydrate count of 30g, and has a dietary fiber count of 2g; your net carbohydrate intake will be 28g. But, if you buy bread that has a total carbohydrate count of 30g, and has a dietary fiber count of 18g, then your net carbohydrate intake will be just 12g (30g – 18g =12g). Since our body does not assimilate the fiber, all it counts it is the net carbohydrate intake.

It is important to read the labels on the foods we buy! On television the other day, a doctor was promoting his book on how to eat healthy. He was recommending for instance whole grain cereals, over regular cereal. He was right, whole grain cereal it is a healthier alternative. But, when it comes to making healthy choices, there is more to consider like carbohydrates, sugar and fiber content as well as fat content. Don't be fooled, read labels always, and look for lower carbohydrate, sugar, and fat content, and high fiber content.

C. Proteins

There are a number of diets on the market, which are both contradictory and confusing. Also, there is a wide spectrum, from no protein diets to high protein diets. If you take the time to actually read them, you will find that they all have facts to sustain their viewpoint. Then of course, you might end up like me, asking yourself, *which one is right?*

When we say the word protein, most likely we envision juicy steaks, roasted chicken, or steamed lobster tail. *"But what are proteins? Do we really need them, and if so, how much do we need?"* Bear with me once more, because knowing is the only way we can make the right choices. Proteins are more complex and larger than carbohydrates or fat molecules. They differ in the fact that they contain nitrogen in addition to carbon, hydrogen, and oxygen.

Approximately 15 to 20 percent of the human body is protein, and that protein exists in many forms. Proteins are the building blocks of tissue, and form a vital part of the nucleus and membranes of the cells. Also, all enzymes (which help the body digest food) found in the body are proteins. Proteins are an important constituent of the blood, like hemoglobin, which transports oxygen from the lungs to the tissues, and carbon dioxide from the tissue back to the lungs. Another form of blood protein is found in the form of antibodies, which is our defense against diseases.

The basic structural units of proteins are *amino acids*. There are approximately 22 known amino acids, 10 referred to as essential amino acids, because they cannot be synthesized within the body. It is important to understand the *quality* of proteins in order to have a proper diet. According to specialists "the efficiency with which a protein is used for growth or maintenance is a measure of its quality" (Joint FAO/WHO Ad Hoc Expert Committee, Geneva, 1973). An ideal protein has a specific pattern of optimal proportions of essential amino acids. If one or more amino acids have less than optimal proportion, the amino acid is designated as "limiting" and adjustments must be made in the diet. For instance, vegetable proteins often have limiting amino acids.

Another way to classify proteins is as complete proteins or partially incomplete proteins.

Complete proteins are those foods that contain all the essential amino acids, in significant amounts and in the proportion needed to maintain life and support growth. They are also referred to as having "high biological value."

Partially incomplete proteins are those foods that contain amino acids in amounts and proportions that may maintain life but not support growth.

The body's demand for protein remains fairly constant, but can vary as a result of certain stress, training periods for sport events, or recovering from debilitating illness, when the protein intake is higher. The recommended daily allowance for protein is 0.8g/K/day. Animal sources of protein, such as milk, eggs, cheese, meat, and poultry, supply proteins of high biological value. Cereals and vegetables are secondary sources of protein in the diet. These are considered partially incomplete proteins. There is wide variation in the biological value of specific food sources of incomplete proteins. For instance, nuts, grains, and legumes all contain more amino acids than fruits and vegetables.

No one will take the time, nor does it seem to make much sense to learn the amino acid content of each food. However, it is important to combine all kinds of protein sources in one's diet to assure the maximum and effective use of the amino acids present in these foods. If diets contain too much protein, beyond the recommended allowance, there is a danger that other important nutrients may be lacking. In addition, if there is an excess of amino acids, the body has no place to store them. It removes and excretes the amino acid group and coverts the reminder of the molecule to glucose, glycogen or fat. Some experiments provide evidence that replacing some of the animal protein with vegetable protein, can reduce the plasma cholesterol.

It has been said, that protein has a hunger controlling effect on the body. We feel fuller faster, which ultimately reduces caloric intake. Moreover, protein helps us burn more calories, since breaking down proteins, takes twice as much energy than breaking down carbohydrates, through the digestion process. Good sources of proteins for a diabetic person are: tuna packed in water, skinless poultry, fish, lean meat, low-fat milk, and low-fat cheese. Animal sources of protein are also good sources of iron, zinc, calcium, riboflavin, vitamins D and B12.

D. Fat

One mention of the word fat is likely to conjure up images of fatty foods, people that are fat, or some personal connection to fat. I believe most of you are as confused as I was about fat. How much of it you should eat if you should eat any, and which ones are good or bad for you. Not everybody knows how fat works biologically. While the terminology is complex, it is not hard to understand fats and how they work.

Fats are composed of the same three elements that are found in carbohydrates: carbon, hydrogen, and oxygen. Fat is a more concentrated form of energy, and contains more carbon and less oxygen then carbohydrates. Biologically fats are referred to as lipids. The main lipids in the body are: triglycerides, phospholipids and cholesterol.

Diabetes is the body's inability to turn food into usable forms of energy. That not only refers to sugar and starches, but to fats also. When insulin is not working properly (Type 2 diabetes), it takes longer than it should to store fat that's just been eaten. This forges the liver to become flooded with fatty acids. In response, the liver emits particles that deposits fat and cholesterol into the blood vessels of the heart, thereby leading to heart problems.

Fat is found in our body in two forms: **structural fat** and **storage fat.** There is a distinction between the two of them. Structural fat is a major component of all cell membranes, internal organs, brain, and nervous tissue. Storage fat is largely saturated fat stored under our skin, abdomens, upper arms, hips, and tights. One of the primary functions of fat is that it constitutes a concentrated form of energy. Also, normal deposits of adipose tissue (storage fat), can protect us from outside forces. This subcutaneous layer insulates the body from rapid changes in environmental temperature, helping to maintain body temperature at a constant level. Adipose tissue it is also deposited around organs like kidneys, and cushions them against any sudden injuries. Fat is, the carrier of the nutrients like vitamins A, D, E, and K.

Cholesterol is an integral part of the cell found in plasma and lymph. Also, along with calcium it may have a role in the tissue repair process. Essential fatty acids seem to regulate cholesterol metabolism. They are important in the maintenance of the function of cellular and sub-cellular membranes in tissue metabolism.

With fat having an important role in one's diet, knowing which ones you do or don't need is very important for your health. All natural fats are mixtures of saturated fats (SFA), monounsaturated fats (MUFA), and polyunsaturated fatty acids (PUFA), depending on the predominant fatty acid type. Healthy fat nutrition requires a balanced intake of these three types in minimally processed form.

Saturated fatty acids (SFA) have no double bounds in the carbon chain, and are solid at room temperature. High amounts of saturated fat are not healthy, and tend to increase the risk for diabetes and cardiovascular disease. Dietary saturated fat, more so than dietary cholesterol, is known to increase blood cholesterol levels. Saturated fat is found mostly in foods such as beef, beef fat, veal, lamb, pork, lard, poultry fat, butter, cream, milk, cheeses, and other dairy products made from whole milk. They are also found in coconut oil, palm oil, cocoa butter and macadamia nuts.

Monounsaturated fatty acids (MUFA) have a single double bond in the carbon chain. They are liquid at room temperature, but partially crystallized and thicken upon refrigeration. Oleic acid is the most common form of monounsaturated fatty acids, and is present in all vegetables oils. Olive oil, peanut oil and sesame oil are rich sources of oleic acid. Also, avocados, pecans, almonds, walnuts, hazelnuts and pistachio contain oleic acid.

Polyunsaturated fatty acids (PUFA) are essential to our metabolism, since mammals cannot create them naturally, like saturated and monounsaturated fats. Like vitamins, PUFA is necessary to sustain human life.

Trans fats are a special type of polyunsaturated fat, and should be minimized or avoided. This is mainly because in terms of metabolism and health, they act more like saturated fats. Trans fats are found in margarine, shortening, candies, crackers, chips, and deep frying oils. Trans fats were originally designed for candle wax. Commercial frying oils are first partially hydrogenated to stabilize them. With trans fats, the food industry can cheaply produce food using hydrogenated oil (a trans fat), while preserving taste, spread ability, and an extended shelf life. During the process of hydrogenation, omega 3 fats, that are healthier but fragile, are destroyed.

Which Ones and How Much?

As I mentioned, trans fats should be avoided. Eating foods that contain trans fats can lead to abnormalities in cholesterol, by decreasing the good and increasing the bad cholesterol. It can increase inflammation and damage to the arterial cells, which make them more prone to clotting.

Polyunsaturated fatty acids are conventionally defined in nutrition texts as linoleic acid and alpha-linoleic acid, both with 18 carbons in the fatty acid chain. Linoleic acid (LA), commonly known as omega 6, is the head for the n-6 PUFA family. Alpha-linoleic acid (LNA), commonly known as omega 3, is the head for the n-3 PUFA family.

Omega 3 fatty acids (n-3PUFA) are necessary to sustain human life. It is believed that omega 3 may help drop excess pounds, regulate blood sugar levels, regulate hunger, aid in reducing cholesterol levels, and help burn more calories by increasing the metabolic rate. Both, linoleic and alpha-linoleic acids are converted by enzymes in our body into more biochemically active long chain forms, known as LC-PUFA derivatives. Diabetics have a strongly impaired ability to make these conversions.

Obtaining a balance between omega-3 and omega-6 fatty acids is essential. Current dietary guidelines have been set by government health agencies, for the overall ratio of dietary omega 6 to omega 3 with ranges from 4:1 to 10:1. Many researchers recommend a ratio 4:1 to 1:1. Human brain tissue contains an omega 6 to omega 3 ratio of around 1:1, while most other cells in the body contain a ratio of 3 to 5:1.

Deficiencies in PUFA and/or excessive unbalanced omega-6 intake, as well as metabolic abnormalities can contribute to chronic and acute diseases, such as diabetes, cardiovascular disease, asthma, allergies, dermatitis, learning disabilities, and multiple sclerosis.

PUFA balance is imperative for both, to balance our hormone production, and for the insulin to act effectively. Cell membranes that are flexible have more and better insulin receptors, allowing for better glucose metabolism. According to the scientists, PUFA helps make cell membrane flexible and SFA makes them stiffer. It has been shown that the cell membrane of a diabetic has an abnormal fat composition: the membranes are too stiff and the levels LC-PUFA are too low. Experiments have shown that increasing membrane flexibility by feeding higher levels of PUFA, but most importantly omega-3, increases the numbers of insulin receptors and insulin action.

Diets high in SFA, trans-fats, and omega-6 opposingly affect insulin efficiency and glucose response. High-fat diets increase the accumulation of storage fat in the skeletal muscles, the major user of the glucose in the body, which are constantly stimulated by insulin. This storage fat leads directly to insulin resistance. Losing some of this fat improves or may even prevent diabetes. It is known that omega-3 reduces stress by dropping the cortisol levels (the stress hormone) and increasing the anti-cortisol levels, while also improving the heart rate.

Conclusion

I had my own proof that this was true. The reason that my husband's sugar level, cholesterol and triglycerides went down after the first month on the diet, was because he was metabolizing foods better than before. In other words, he actually improved his insulin efficiency and the glucose response. He accomplished this by daily exercise, and increase in his omega-3 intake by having fish 3-4 times a week. Also, by eliminating the trans fats from his diet, and reducing the SFA intake.

In order to improve the ratio between omega-6 and omega-3, fried foods, corn oil, safflower, sunflower, peanut, and sesame oil should be avoided. Cold-pressed olive oil and canola oil should be used instead. Also, the intake of leafy green vegetables, nuts, navy beans, and flaxseeds should be increased.

Good sources of omega-6 are: flax, pumpkin, sunflower, sesame, and grape seeds. Also walnuts, peanuts, pecans, almonds, soybeans, wheat germs, safflower, and rice bran are good sources as well. Omega-3 is found in significant quantities in flax, mustard, canola, hemp, and grape seeds, walnuts, and soybeans, and at a low level in green leafy vegetables. Oils containing omega-3 should be consumed cold-pressed and unrefined, as in salads or baking. Those oils are not suitable for stove-top cooking and deep frying.

Good sources of omega-3 derivatives are found mainly in cold water fatty marine fish, such as salmon, herring, sardines, fresh tuna, mackerel, sturgeon, bluefish, and halibut. The products with the highest omega-3 content come from animals that primarily have grass diet. For instance, organic eggs from grass-fed chickens have lower levels of saturated fat, since grains force the bird's bodies to increase the insulin levels. According to the specialists, having a diet that contains balanced unrefined PUFA is the only way to cure persistent cravings for fatty foods. In addition, it results in the loss of body's storage fat.

Low-fat and fat-free diets are very popular these days. Media continues to educate us about the risks of high-fat diets, while providing low-fat cooking tips and recipes. However, it is possible to do more harm than good with diets that are low in fat, because our immune, digestive, cardiovascular, and neurological systems are all dependent on PUFA, along with our skin. It has been said that without a balanced PUFA intake, we can never look or feel our best. Neither will our bodies be able to defend from diseases, environmental toxins, or premature aging.

Today, there are many farms for both birds and animals that sell organic meat, eggs, milk, and dairy products. Organic food is by far a healthier alternative, since most of the meats found in grocery stores come from grain or corn-fed animals that are pumped-up to make fattier and tastier cuts. It is known that wild game has about 4% fat, while most commercially available beef contain about nine times that amount. There are many stores that now sell organic products. Though the organic foods are higher in price than the regular ones, including the organic foods into your diet will save you money in a long run. Avoiding illnesses, improving health, longevity, and the quality of life has no price tag.

E. Vitamins and Minerals

Most of us have vitamins in our cabinet. We've come to learn that they are important for our health, and they should be part of our daily diet. There is a wide variety of vitamins and minerals supplements on the market, and are taken by both adults and children alike. But what exactly are vitamins?

Vitamins are nutrients. They serve as part of enzymes or coenzymes that are essential for life. Vitamins are a group of organic compounds that are essential in small quantities for the normal metabolism of nutrients. The role of vitamins in human nutrition is divided in two categories: prevention of disease and participation in the regulation of body process.

Vitamins do not yield energy. They are either classified as water-soluble or fat-soluble. Water-soluble vitamins, such as Vitamin C (ascorbic acid) and B-complex, are not stored in the body, and therefore must be constantly supplied in our diet. Fat-soluble vitamins, such as Vitamins A, D, E, and K, are stored in the body primarily in the liver, but also in the fatty tissue. Excessive accumulation of these vitamins can be toxic. Some of the richest sources of vitamins are green leafy vegetables, whole grains, skim milk, nuts, seeds, lean meats, poultry, and citrus fruits.

Minerals

Minerals are inorganic compounds found in the body that are vital for proper bodily function. Their categorization as major minerals, or trace minerals is based on the amount that are needed daily. We require a *minimum* of 100 milligrams (mg) per day of the following **major minerals:** calcium, chloride, magnesium, phosphorus, potassium, sodium, and sulfur. We only require a *maximum* of 100 milligrams per day of the following **trace minerals:** copper, fluoride, iodine, iron, magnesium, selenium, and zinc.

In general, minerals have two main functions. First, minerals are a constituent of the body in both hard and soft tissue. For instance, calcium, magnesium, and phosphorus are very important in the structure of bones and teeth. While other minerals on the other hand, are involved in the structure of the body. Examples of this are such as iodine in the thyroid gland and its excretion, magnesium in the muscles and blood. Potassium is also an integral part of the muscles and other organs.

Many of the hormones, enzymes, and other aspects of body composition include minerals in their makeup. Every body's cell makes a continuous demand for minerals. For instance, iron and phosphorus are found in every living cell. Minerals in the cell influence the vital process of oxidation, secretion, and growth. The supply of minerals in the cell may preclude or facilitate the process of cellular metabolism or metabolic homeostasis. In their next important role, minerals act as regulators and are necessary to sustain body functions, like the functioning of nerves. If the concentration of calcium, magnesium, sodium, and potassium in the fluids bathing the nerve cell is altered, the ability to transmit nerve impulses will be disrupted. The functioning and even the survival of body cell depend on the maintenance of body neutrality. The maintenance of acid-base balance neutrality is related to some minerals. Also, minerals contribute to the water and electrolyte balance of the body.

Plant foods are good sources for many of the trace minerals. Animal products, mainly seafood, are the best sources of most minerals, because animals eat plants year after year. This thereby allows minerals from the plants to become concentrated in the animal tissue.

Antioxidants

Antioxidants include: vitamin C, vitamin E, and beta-carotene which is a vitamin A precursor (provitamin), selenium, zinc, and numerous botanical products like grape seeds, pine bark, green tea, and rosemary. Antioxidants are synergetic, and work best when they are all supplemented together.

Antioxidants are nutrients that help to prevent damage caused by molecular particles called free radicals. Numerous studies showed that diets high in antioxidants help reduce the risk for cancer, heart disease, and stroke. Also, adequate supplemental levels of antioxidants, may directly improve glucose tolerance and insulin sensitivity. Antioxidants are responsible for the detoxification of potentially damaging free radicals and the reduction of inflammation. The most noted nutritional antioxidants are: vitamin F, vitamin C, and beta-carotene. The daily requirement of vitamins, minerals, and antioxidants is different for diabetics than for non-diabetics. Check with your doctor to establish the adequate daily dosage that is right for you.

Chapter Four

KNOWING YOUR BODY

We all know our body, or we think we do. We see it every day, we admire or criticize it. But do we really know what is inside of the outside image? Do we really know how our body functions, what are its needs, what is the process that takes place inside? In the same way, we all heard about cholesterol, blood pressure, and body weight. But do we really understand what we think we know? Well this chapter will do just that. It will help you understand your body and its functions, as a first step in achieving a better health. You cannot fix what you don't know.

What is Inflammation

Inflammation is a chemical reaction that happens within the bloodstream, as a result of the oxygen-free radicals becoming oxidized. Inflammation can also be caused by food allergies such as lactose intolerance, or allergies to gluten. Bodily example of inflammation can range from the way in which the liver responds to saturated and trans-fats, to the way in which the body responds to toxins from smoke and stress. The inflammatory response can cause hypertension, high cholesterol, and insulin resistance. The more inflammation we have in our intestines, the easier it is for toxins to enter the bloodstream. This in turn, lowers our body's efficiency of processing food calories, which results in us feeling worse.

What is cholesterol?

Cholesterol is a waxy substance produced by the liver, and is found among the lipids in the bloodstream, as well as in all the body's cells. Cholesterol can also be found in foods like meats, egg yolks, shellfish, and whole milk dairy products.

Our body needs cholesterol to function, to form cell membranes and create hormones. When too much cholesterol is made or absorbed from the foods we eat, it gets deposited along the walls of the arteries, where it combines with other substances to form plaque. Plaque is dangerous because it raises blood pressure by making the heart work harder to pump blood through the narrowed vessels. It is also dangerous because, plaque can break off and get into the bloodstream where it forms clots, which eventually leads to stroke, heart attack, paralysis and death.

The three main types of cholesterol are:

- LDL(low-density lipoproteins)
- HDL(high-density lipoproteins)
- VLDL(very low-density lipoproteins)

LDL cholesterol also known as "bad cholesterol" typically contains 60 to70 percent of the total serum cholesterol, and is associated with the risk of coronary heart disease. One function of the LDL is to supply cholesterol to cells for synthesis of cell membranes, and steroid hormones. Exposure of LDL to the cells that make up the innermost lining of the arteries can result in its oxidation. This can lead to the accumulation of cholesterol and to the formation of atherosclerotic plaque.

HDL it is known as the "good cholesterol" because it actually helps remove bad cholesterol from the body by carrying it back to the liver, where it's passed from the body. Some experts believe that HDL removes excess cholesterol from plaque and thus slows down its growth. High level of HDL seems to protect against heart attacks.

VLDL contains a type of fat called triglycerides, and like high cholesterol, high triglycerides generates the risk of heart disease.

High levels of cholesterol (over 200mg/dL), are unhealthy and indicates a greater risk for atherosclerosis and heart attack. The important factor here is the ratio between LDL/HDL. Ideal level of HDL should be between 40 and 59 mg/dL (milligram/ deciliter), and LDL levels under 160mg/dL.

While these days there are a lot of medications to assist in lowering cholesterol levels, it is best to naturally control cholesterol levels within the diet. How? Here are few facts:

- Eliminating the bad fats and increasing the good ones, will help reduce the cholesterol level.

- The B vitamin called niacin, grapefruit, and oat bran all lower the LDL cholesterol level.

- Niacin, also like cranberries increases the HDL cholesterol.

- Garlic lowers total cholesterol level, and possibly help limit damage to the heart after a heart attack.

❖ Appendix 3 will list all the foods known to have an effect on controlling cholesterol level.

What is Blood Pressure?

Regardless of our reason for seeing the doctor, our blood pressure is usually one of the first things checked upon arriving at the doctor's office. In most cases, and certainly in my case, I was never given the results of the reading unless I asked. I am not sure why, perhaps doctors don't think patients will understand the numbers. In my husband's case, when we were told that his blood pressure was high, and that we need to control it, we were at a lost as to what to do first.

This is why I believe that it's important to know and understand what blood pressure is, in order to know how to control it. These days, we can monitor our blood pressure very closely, since we can take it almost anywhere at no cost.

Scientifically, blood pressure is the pressure exerted by the blood against the inside of the arterial walls. It is the force that moves the blood through the circulatory system, and is measured through the systolic and diastolic pressure. The systolic pressure is the pressure being exerted when the heart contracts, and it is symbolized by the top number in the reading. While, diastolic pressure, is the pressure in the arteries when the heart is at rest, and it is symbolized by the bottom number on the reading.

The ideal blood pressure should be 120/80.

High blood pressure, or "hypertension," happens when systolic and/or diastolic pressure is elevated. Resistance to the blood flow is caused by friction between the blood and the walls of the blood vessels—*the grater the friction, the greater the resistance to the flow.*

Vascular friction depends on the thickness of the blood, the length, and the diameter of the blood vessel.

Atherosclerosis is a slow and progressive disease. It involves the narrowing of the lumen of the arteries, which is caused by fatty substances, calcium, and collagen, as well as other cellular materials. These materials are deposited as a plaque-like material on the inside walls of the arteries. The arteries become stiff and hardened. The action most responsible for a heart attack is plaque thrombosis (blood clots formation), which usually occurs when plaque is fissuring, tearing, or rupturing.

Some of the many factors that raise blood pressure are stress, high levels of sodium, and lack of calcium or potassium. Physical inactivity is one of the things that lead to being overweight, and being overweight leads to high blood pressure.

Hypertension (high blood pressure) can also cause plaque build-up in one of the brain's arteries, eventually cutting off the blood flow. Kidney failure or heart attack can also follow from dangerous plaque accumulation.

Fortunately, to lower or control the blood pressure isn't hard. Scientific studies show that:

- Potassium helps to lower the blood pressure by eliminating excess sodium from the circulatory system. This causes the blood vessels to dilate.

- Lowering the sodium consumption by including low-sodium foods in the diet, cooking with no salt or with salt substitute, also helps to lower the blood pressure.

- Increasing physical activity and including certain foods in the diet, will contribute to lowering and controlling the blood pressure.

  ❖ Appendix 3 will list all the vegetables and fruits known to have an effect on lowering blood pressure.

Obesity and Central Obesity

When we see such diseases as diabetes, coronary heart disease, psychological disturbances, kidney disease, hypertension, strokes, liver and biomechanical ailments, they all have one enemy in common—*obesity*. I used to think that only significantly overweight people (those with visibly larger bodies) were considered obese. But, after much research, way of thinking changed.

Experts believe that the normal body weight attained between the ages 25 to30 should be maintained for life. A high waist-to-hip circumference ratio is used as an indicator of intra-abdominal or "central" fat distribution. This pattern of fat distribution is considered to carry more risk for diseases than a low-ratio, which indicates a "peripheral" fat distribution. This presents less of a risk for metabolic disorders.

What is Your Body Shape?

We all tend to want the "model-type" bodies, but unfortunately some of us have big bellies and hips to deal with. Due to the **hypothalamus** gland,— located in the center of the brain—we are shaped differently. It is responsible for the control of many body functions, and determines where the body stores fat. It is the master gland that also regulates the metabolism.

I remember my husband once telling me that he became a diabetic when he quit smoking, due to the metabolic changes that occurred. Though I thought the real reason was that he couldn't control his appetite, and ate too much, I never told him differently. I eventually learned that we were somehow both right.

Throughout life, a person's hypothalamus can become seriously overtaxed. Hypothalamus contains a mechanism that initiates eating and another mechanism that deters overeating. If small lesions are induced in those areas of hypothalamus, the changes in our eating patterns could be quite dramatic. The same effects could occur as a result of traumatic or stressful event.

This has to be the explanation as to why and how my father became a diabetic. He was in a hospital for two weeks with pneumonia. There was fluid in both of his lungs. It took sometimes strong treatment, but eventually he got better. And, though he was only 44 years of age, physically active, and in great shape, he was still shortly thereafter, diagnosed with Type 2 diabetes.

Consumption of massive amounts of calories in a short period of time will also cause the hypothalamus to function abnormally resulting in a low metabolic rate, intense and constant hunger, and the storing of the fat in the secure fat reserve in the belly area. This belly fat is called **omentum.**

While in no way trying to overload you with big names that are difficult to remember, it is critical to know and understand how central obesity contributes to diabetes.

Omentum

Omentum is a fatty layer of tissue located behind the abdominal wall, underneath the muscles of the stomach. It surrounds the internal organs, providing them with the best energy source. Omentum fat contributes to Type 2 diabetes, by making it difficult for the insulin to deliver glucose inside the cells. As a result, this leaves the glucose to float around in the blood. Also, omentum fat uses the insulin, which hinders it from doing its job. This contributes to high glucose levels which:

- Prevents white blood cells from fighting infections.
- Weakens the immune system.
- Keeps oxygen from getting to the tissue.
- Attaches to the proteins in the blood and in the tissue.

This can lead to development of cataracts, joint abnormalities, lung problems, and nerve damage in parts of the body furthest from the brain, including the hands and feet.

It is also said, that psychological factors may play a role in obesity. People often overeat to obtain certain satisfactions, or some overeat to compensate for certain personality flaws or deficits. An individual may also overeat due to their strong cues toward certain foods. Unusual eating patterns such as eating little to no breakfast or lunch, and then consuming large meal in the evening can lead to obesity. Binge eating is another eating pattern that can also lead to obesity.

While there are genetic influences that contribute to particular body types, or behaviors, I've learned that this can be curved by making healthy decisions and eating the right foods.

Body Weight Control

There are many reasons we eat other than hunger satisfaction. Some of these reasons are prompted by social events such holidays, celebrations and other gatherings. Other reasons may have emotional roots such as eliminating stress, or reacting to a specific life event. There is however, only one reason why any of us actually need food and that is for the energy it supplies to the body.

Type 2 diabetes is a metabolic condition, whereby the body is unable to properly process what we eat. Metabolism literally means "change." It is the rate at which our body burns the calories that we eat.

Calories

The term "calories" is becoming more and more popular these days. We hear it every day in television commercials, food advertising, weight control programs, and even on food labels. Counting calories is becoming a common practice, but it's a practice that I find unreasonable to follow. Having half of a chocolate bar or half of a bagel, just because I met my calories intake is hard and often unsatisfying. We're almost forced to either eat none of it, or all of it.

This is why I came up with some recipes for desserts that are not bad for a diabetic to have. I've also found that making desserts in small portions and storing them in separate containers, which are out of sight, really helps. We all know the old adage, "Out of sight—out of mind." From calories standpoint, my husband should be very happy as his diet does not require him to count calories. He restricted his daily menu to recommended amounts of lean protein, low-fat dairy products, good fats, and plenty of low-calories foods (vegetables).

What are Calories?

Since there is so much discussion about calories, it is only reasonable to discuss what they actually are, and why they are important.

Calories in foods are a measure of the amount of energy supplied to the individual by the diet. They are also referred to in the scientific term as "kilocalorie." The energy requirement of an individual, also expressed in calories, refer to the amount of energy a person needs to live and work. We need energy for our organs to function, our muscles to move, and our bodies to keep warm.

The energy that we consume and store is primarily used to power the anatomical system and structures. The human body requires a sufficient amount of energy from food for: basal metabolism, the synthesis of body tissue that naturally occurs in growth and maintenance, for physical activity, heat regulation, excretory processes, and for physiological and psychological stress.

Basal metabolism is the energy metabolism of the body at complete rest, in a comfortable position, comfortably warm, mentally and physically relaxed. It is the energy required to perform normal body functions including respiratory, circulatory, tissue maintenance, cellular metabolism, glandular activity, and maintenance of muscles tone.

It is great to know that due to the basal metabolism, our bodies are constantly in motion and we burn calories while we watch T.V., read our favorite book, or even sleep. In fact, 60 to 80 percent of our daily calories are burned through basal metabolism, which requires no exertion on our part. Another 10 to 30 percent of our calories are burned through digestion and 10 to15 percent is burned through physical activity. Keep in mind that all movement speeds up metabolism. For instance, an increase in body temperature of just one degree increases the metabolic rate by 14%.

How Much Food Do We Need?

For body weight to remain constant, food intake must equal the energy needs. We gain weight when too much food is consumed, but not being burned. If our energy needs exceed the energy produced by the food we eat, we then lose weight. In this case, the body consumes its own fat, and then protein, which results in a loss of body weight. The caloric deficit should represent both an increased expenditure of energy through physical activity, and a controlled reduced caloric intake.

If you prefer to count calories, it is important to know your daily caloric needs. The method I've found most helpful is the one presented by Ross and Jackson, (Ross, R.M. and J. S. Jackson, 1990) for my husband and me.

Their formula states that daily caloric need = **BEE + GA + EX,**
Where: **BEE** represents basal energy expenditure
GA represents general activity (or basal metabolism)
EX represents energy cost of exercise
Their formula varies for man and women, and is elaborate below:

Males: BEE= 66+ (13.7x Wt) + (5xHt) - (6.9x A)

Females: BEE= 665= (9.6xWt) + (1.7xHt) - (4.7xA)

Where: **Wt**= weight in kilograms, **Ht**= height in centimeters, and **A**= age in years

Knowing the energy cost of exercise, is not important unless you are one of those people like my daughter, who, after she eats a slice of cake, will go run for 30 minutes, just to burn it off. If counting calories is your thing, it is important to know that both 1 gram of protein and 1 gram of carbohydrates are equal to 4 calories, and 1 gram of fat is equal to 7 calories. This helps you to make adjustments according to your daily caloric intake.

Since obesity is specific for Type 2 diabetes, keeping weight under control at an optimal level is essential. I found this very easy to do by following a healthy diet, and being active. This is why it is very important to know our foods and their contribution to our health, since different foods create different insulin response.

Foods with high levels of simple carbohydrates like white bread, pasta and white rice, cereals and fruits with a high sugar content and low levels of fiber, increases the glucose level into the bloodstream shortly after eating. This in turn due their fast digestion and absorption causes the insulin levels to spike, by working quickly to turn that blood sugar into fat. In the case of Type2 diabetes, when insulin resistance had already occurred, insulin cannot do its job, and that sugar stays into the bloodstream, not being able to enter and feed the cells. Dairy products such as milk and yogurt, also creates insulin surges, but without the corresponding effect on blood sugar level. When the blood sugar level remains relatively constant, and within normal ranges, it allows insulin to do its job, by using the nutrients in the bloodstream to build and repair cells, muscles, tissue, etc. Continuing to flood the bloodstream with high levels of sugar triggers high levels of insulin, which trains the body to eventually become less efficient to insulin, creating insulin resistance.

How does the body actually process what we eat? The digestion process is affected largely by the types of foods that we eat. An explanation follows for each group.

Simple carbohydrates/simple sugars such as table sugar, fructose and lactose are quickly absorbed and sent to the liver, where a digestion process takes place, and the liver tells the body to convert that sugar into fat if it cannot be used *immediately* for energy.

Complex carbohydrates such as cereal grains, rice, roots, fiber, oat bran, beans, fruits and vegetables take longer to digest. However if the body cannot use it for energy when it is release, it gets converted into fat.

Protein found in meat, eggs, and beans, just to name a few, are broken down into small amino acids, which are sent to the liver. If the liver cannot send them to the muscles, they get converted to glucose, and eventually fat when not used for energy.

Fat gets broken down into smaller particles that are absorbed as fat. Good fats like those found in fish and nuts decrease the body's inflammatory response, while bad fats increase it.

Hungry or Full?

Our hypothalamus, represents a key command center, and contains the satiety center. This center is controlled by two chemicals: one increases metabolism and reduces appetite, while the other, decreases metabolism and increases appetite.

There is enough evidence to suggest that there are two hormones that influence our hunger and satiety level. The hormone *leptin* is a protein secreted by stored fat that sends signals to the satiety center to make us feel full and satisfied. The stimulation of leptin shuts off hunger and stimulates us to burn more calories. By losing weight, the cells become more sensitive to leptin. On the other hand, *ghrelin* is the hormone that makes us want to eat, and it is secreted by our stomach and intestines when the stomach is empty. When the stomach is full, the levels of ghrelin are reduced, which in turn reduces the appetite.

Stomach growling stimulates the appetite, making us feel hungry. This is our stomach's way of telling us to eat, but unfortunately, it doesn't tell us how much to eat. Eating smaller portions satisfies our hunger with a lot less calorie intake. Eating the right foods such as good fats, lean protein and complex carbohydrates, will keep hormones in balance and keep us satisfied. While eating the wrong foods such as simple sugars, disturbs our body's hormone levels, by constantly sending the signal that we are hungry, and thereby making it difficult to satisfy our appetite.

Protein and fiber with high water content have a great effect on satiety, whereas simple carbohydrates have the least effect. Fiber slows down digestion and keeps our stomach full for a longer time, which gives us a greater feeling of satiety, and an increase of appetite suppressing. Fiber also controls sugar levels, while decreasing insulin levels. Studies show that consuming fiber in the morning makes us less hungry in the afternoon. The satiety effect of fat is similar to that of protein and fiber.

From the standpoint of converting calories, our body processes fat most efficiently, since the body does not need to expend too many calories to store it, this results in us keeping more of it. While on the other hand, our body works hard to process proteins, thus burning more calories. The way food influence our satiety center dictates whether we should eat more or less food.

Our Genetic Make-up

Like me, you're probably wondering how some people can primarily eat fast foods all the time, and yet remain thin. In my research, I learned that some people can have a bad genetic response to good diets, while other people can have a good genetic response to bad diets. Glands which make up the endocrine system and produce our hormones are responsible for the genetic conditions that could influence metabolism and weight.

The primary glands are:

1. **Thyroid gland:** thyroid hormones influences how quickly or slowly we burn energy.

2. **Adrenal glands:** when chronically stressed they produce cortisol, and cortisol inhibits. High cortisol levels, reduces insulin sensitivity. The kidney also responds to high cortisol levels, by retaining water and salt, which increases blood pressure.

3. **Pancreas:** secrets insulin; the substance that helps the glucose travel from the blood into the cells. Insulin has a mechanism that tells us to eat less. But when insulin resistance occurs in the cells, it negates the appetite-control effect, and we continue to eat.

There are a total of nine known hormones that make us eat more, and fourteen hormones that make us eat less. When hormones don't work normally, the only solution is to reprogram the hormonal circuitry by eating the right foods. I was astounded when I learned that one could develop diabetes after years of eating foods that are high in carbohydrates, which are easy to convert into sugar. These include white bread, pasta, potatoes, and white rice. This was surprising to me, being that they were part of our home-cooked meals.

How Much and When to Eat

In addition to the effects of consuming a high-carbohydrates diet, the propensity to develop diabetes is tied in with our metabolism. All of us burn calories at different amounts and different rates. It is important to eat throughout the day in order to reset the metabolic rate and release the fat reserves. In order to lose weight we have to prevent the body from going into starvation mode. When we go for long periods of time without eating, our brain senses starvation, and sends a signal throughout the body to store fat, in order to create a reserve for "famine time."

Physical performance and endurance are also influenced by how often we eat. Studies show that eating 3 meals throughout the day, along with **2 to 3** snacks, improves body performance, versus only eating 3 meals.

Simply put, the less food eaten at one time means the less blood rushing to the stomach, which leaves more blood available for muscles, causing us in turn to feel less tired. After a rich meal we feel tired for a while, and tend to fall into a state of rest "siesta" This is because all the blood rushes to the stomach for digestion, making the rest of the body feel tired. Therefore, in order to lose weight, reduce appetite, and increase physical performance, all of us, especially diabetics, must eat frequent healthy meals and snacks to avoid spikes in insulin secretion.

Eat when you hungry, but remember to eat the "right foods." Also remember, "Don't overeat, but don't under eat." These guidelines will help you to reprogram your body to work the way it's suppose to work.

———— Chapter Five ————

KNOWING YOUR FOODS

Most of us become familiar with food groups and food pyramid at an early age. I believe food pyramids are a great tool for teaching children to eat healthy, especially with such a high percentage of obese children. Visual clues play an important role in making selections, which is why the advertising business makes a lot of money. Also, knowing the nutrients in different food groups helps us to select an optimal diet, and make smarter choices such as reaching for an apple instead of a bagel. Knowing this information will also help save lots of money in the long run, being that we won't be as quick to believe and buy everything that is seen on television commercials and ads. Knowing our foods is the key in helping us design a diet that's right for us.

1. Milk and Milk Products

Since the earliest days of civilization, milk has been used as an important food for humans. As children, many of us drank a glass of milk at least once a day, whether it was cold or warm (in my country, we prefer it warm) with cookies, cakes, bread, cereal or by itself. Some of us still include milk in our diets as adults. But, the question none of us have really asked is, "Do we really need milk?"

I came across many opinions regarding the inclusion of milk in our diets. I believe that milk is a keeper. The greatest contribution of milk from a nutrition point of view is *calcium,* which is very poorly distributed among other foods. When calcium needs are not met by food, the body must resort to drawing calcium from the bones of the body. The protein in milk is of unusually high quality. Milk is also known for its significant contribution of vitamin A and riboflavin. The main carbohydrate in milk is lactose, which is a milk sugar, and averages about 4.8% in whole cow's milk. For a diabetic, however, it is best to choose 2% milk or skim milk, in order to reduce the fat in the diet. Skim milk has most of the fat removed, and is lower in calories and vitamin A (unless it is fortified), but the calcium content remains the same. It is important to read the individual labels on milk products that you choose because oftentimes, when fat is extracted, the sugar content increases. The best milk that I've found on the market for a diabetic diet is "Hood Calorie Countdown," which has only *5 grams of fat, 5 grams of carbohydrates and 3 grams of sugar.*

Another good source of calcium is yogurt. Yogurt has the nutritional value of whole milk unless the preparation method alters it. I recommend making your own yogurt. This way, you will know exactly what's in it. Also watch out for nondairy products such as whipped toppings, coffee creamers, and imitation sour cream, because these are made with saturated fats such as coconut oil or partially hydrogenated oils. These products are definitely not healthy for anyone, and are not recommended for low or restricted-fat diets, or diabetic diets.

Cheese is another milk product. It varies in nutritional value based on the type of milk used, the amount of moisture, and the preparation of the cheese. Choosing low-fat and low-sodium options, which are still nutritious is the right choice for a diabetic person.

2. Vegetables, Fruits, Legumes, Seeds and Nuts

Next on the list are vegetable, which are also a good source of calcium. The best thing about the fruit and vegetable group is that they are low in calories. Generally, a 100 gram (½ cup) portion of fruit or vegetables does not exceed 100 calories. Foods in this group that are higher in calories contain immature seeds such as peas and lima beans. Starchy roots or tubers such as potatoes, sweet potatoes, and bananas, are high in sugar. With the exception of green leaf vegetables, and those foods that contain immature seeds, this food group tends to be low in protein value, and needs to be supplemented with animal protein to have a higher biological value. These foods are also a rich source of certain minerals. The green colored parts of plants, including the leaves, are an excellent source of iron such as beet greens, dandelion greens, kale, chard, spinach, and broccoli.

Two characteristics of vegetables play an important role in determining their nutrition value: color and the part of the plant that it is eaten. For instance, leaves and stems such as lettuce, asparagus, and kale are rich sources of vitamin A, C, and iron. Deep-yellow and dark green vegetables provide a superior contribution of vitamin A to one's daily diet. Vegetables such as broccoli, cabbage, tomatoes, green peppers, salad greens, mustard greens, and turnips are rich in vitamin C.

One of the questions I thought about, was "Why should we choose sweet potatoes over white potatoes?" Although sweet potatoes contain more calories than white potatoes, they are lower in carbohydrate content, and provide 8100 IU of vitamin A per 100 grams, while white potatoes have only trace amounts of vitamin A.

Fruits also represent a good source of vitamins. Several fruits like prunes, raw cantaloupe, raw apricots, and watermelon contain vitamin A. Although they are not rich sources, some fruits do contribute calcium and iron. Orange juice is a good source of calcium, and prunes contain some iron. High values of vitamin C can be found in citrus fruit, with the highest amount being found in fresh oranges. This provides as much as 60 milligrams of ascorbic acid in each. The same amount of ascorbic acid can be derived from eating 2/3 of a cup of strawberries. Vitamin C (ascorbic acid), which is a strong water-soluble antioxidant, helps aid in the regulation of intercellular oxidation-reduction potentials. It also helps protect other antioxidants, such as vitamin A and E, and the essential fatty acids.

Antioxidants also help to improve glucose tolerance and insulin sensitivity. When choosing fruits for my husband's diet, I take into consideration both, the nutrition value as well as the amount of carbohydrates or sugar contained in each, making sure to keep the sugar in low amounts.

All fruits and vegetables contain considerable amounts of fiber, but the amount of it varies by the portion of the plant that is eaten. For instance, tubers such as potatoes have little fiber, whereas celery stalks and apple skins contain a considerable amount of fiber.

Nuts, because of their high-fat and-low moisture content, are a concentrated food that is high in calories. Most of the commonly eaten nuts will yield 150 to 200 calories per ounce. The protein, found in nuts such as almonds and pecans, is complete. Though their contribution is small when it comes to minerals, vitamin A and vitamin C, they do provide some iron and calcium.

3. Cereal and breads

People all over the world eat grains of some kind. Often times they can be found in breakfast cereals, rice, oats, or pasta. These grains are either whole or partially (enriched). The types of grains eaten vary based on the dietary patterns of one area of the world versus another. Grains have become a major staple of almost everyone's diet.

An important question is, *"Should we have grains in our diet? And if so, in what amounts should we consume them?"*

To answer these questions, we first need to know what they contribute in relation to nutrition. It is important to know whether the whole grain, or only a part of the grain was used, and whether the food has been enriched.

The preparation of the grain affects the nutrition value. When part or all of the bran is removed, as in the case of white rice or flour, the nutrition value is greatly reduced. This is because the essential minerals and vitamins such as iron, phosphorus, magnesium, protein, vitamin B6, and thiamin are lost. More importantly, the fiber is lost.

The main contribution of cereals and breads is energy. The required amounts should be based on the amount of energy we consume. However, for a diabetic, the amount should be limited since its consumption can significantly raise the sugar level. I personally love French or Italian style bread. I grew up with it and have come to love its unique taste. But, I've also learned to like other healthier breads such as whole wheat or rye bread. If you must have bread in your diet, there are several choices of healthier breads on the market to choose from, including 98% fat-free, sugar-free, gluten-free, breads made from whole grain, whole wheat or rye.

When it comes to rice, brown rice should be chosen over white rice. This is because brown rice has been milled so that the hull of the grain has been removed but almost all the bran has been retained. This helps maintain the richness in thiamin, vitamin B6, riboflavin, niacin, iron, and protein. You must keep in mind that unless breads and cereals maintain a high percentage of the grain, its only contribution is calories.

4. Meat, fish, poultry and eggs

I don't know about you, but I am a meat lover. I cannot imagine having a meal without meat. With all due respect to vegetarians, I myself know that I am not the vegetarian type. I've also learned in my research that the vegetarian diet it's not necessarily the healthier choice.

Concerning the protein, meat, fish, and poultry are of the greatest sources of complete protein. Meat proteins are adequate for both maintenance and growth and effectively supplement incomplete proteins in the diet. The cuts of meat have no effect on meat's nutritional value. The nutrients found in chuck beef are as adequate as those found in porterhouse steak. However, as the fat increases, other nutrients are diluted.

It is important to remember, the leaner the meat the higher the protein value will be. Also, the higher the fat content, the greater the energy value of meat. While it has been proven, for diabetics or anyone else watching their weight, lean meats are the best choice. With a lower daily recommended protein allowance, smaller servings of meat are encouraged.

Besides the fact that meat contains complete proteins, meat is also rich in phosphorus, magnesium, niacin, riboflavin, and vitamins B6 and B12. It contains practically no vitamin A and very little vitamin C.

Shellfish is especially high in iron, which is responsible for carrying the oxygen in the blood. Most saltwater fish and shellfish are an excellent source of iodine. Fish like tuna and salmon have a high content of omega 3, which has a great influence on reducing stress, by reducing the cortisol level and improving the anti-cortisol.

Eggs are very similar to meat in their nutritional value. Two eggs are equal to one 2-ounces serving of meat in protein value. They are very adequate in protein in both the egg white and the egg yolk. Eggs are an important source of protein for growing children. The egg white is also a rich source of riboflavin. The yolk is one of the best sources of vitamin A, and a good source of vitamins E, B6, and B12.

There is no difference in the nutritional value of eggs from one breed of chicken versus another, nor is the color of the shell an indication of nutritional value. The nutritional value varies based on the food that is given to the hen. Eggs are not a high source of energy, but, they due contribute calories, one egg is approximately 80 calories. The only detriment of eggs is the high cholesterol content; therefore, it is recommended that one's diet be limited to 3-4 eggs per week. Because of the high cholesterol content, I found it beneficial to limit my husband's diet to 2 eggs every other week. There are many available egg substitutes on the market. I chose Egg Beaters for my husband's diet because they contain no cholesterol or fat. The carbohydrates content is only 1%, and most importantly, they have the closest taste to real eggs.

Food Pyramid

Everyone has become more conscientious about eating healthy foods. This can be seen through the abundance of TV infomercial, diet and cooking books that are now on the market. As a result, the food pyramid can be prominently seen almost everywhere you go: doctors' offices, grocery stores, schools, and day care centers. In our introduction to the food pyramid, we were taught to use this as a guideline for healthy eating. We were taught to believe that if we obtained various foods, and followed their recommended serving amount, then we would be eating healthy, right?

I say, not so! The food pyramid is based on the assumption that everyone requires the same foods and that one healthy diet works for everyone. However, because we are genetically and metabolically different, this simply cannot be the case. For instance, the food pyramid recommends a low-fat, high-carbohydrate diet. Based on my observations and trials of various diets with my husband and how they affected his sugar level, I now believe high carbohydrate intake is at the root of diabetes and obesity.

In my research, I learned that not all fats are bad, and that we do in fact need to eat some fats, such as the healthy ones found in cold water fish, nuts, avocado, and olive oil. I learned about the various types of carbohydrates, which ones were good and most needed, and those that needed to be avoided by diabetics and those needing to lose weight. These include some foods such as bread and pasta (especially the white ones), which are both foods we need to limit. I learned the importance of protein, and which meats are good for us. I also learned that overall, we tend to have an over-consumption of grains, perhaps based on our understanding of the food pyramid. Getting educated about nutrition and foods, and the roles that they play in regulating our body's functions, helped me develop a food meal plan that worked for my husband; a meal plan that lowered his sugar level, cholesterol, blood pressure, and triglycerides. The knowledge that I gained through research and experiments (studying foods and their influence on my husband' sugar level), helped me design our own food pyramid.

Until recently, I was always one of the few fortunate people who could eat everything. No matter how much I ate, I remained trim and slim. I had a fast metabolism that allowed me to readily burn what I ate. I know that whatever weight that I gained in the last few years has a lot to do with age. After forty, everything slows down and the required food intake reduces. But, I also know that part of the weight gain has to do with the quality of the food. Almost everything now is genetically modified, quickly grown, and with high contents of hormones, antibiotics and pesticides. I believe that the change in my metabolism and biochemistry could be attributed to these factors.

I remember when I first came to the United States it took me almost a year to adapt to the taste of food. To me, everything simply tasted different than the foods I was used to such as the tomatoes, fruits, and even chicken.

In Romania, I grew up accustomed to the seasonal changes in our eating habits, as well as the food choices. Growing up we ate what was locally grown and in season. Each season had its own type of foods, such as light varieties of meat, if any, and lots of salads in the summer, and heavier meats and citrus fruits in the winter. This way, there was a rotation of foods throughout the year, which I considered to be healthier for us.

As far as I remember, we didn't have that many metabolically related diseases. But, now due to the modern miracles of manufacturing, processing, preserving, and transporting, the food industry has made it possible for us to have any kind of food at any time of the year, anywhere in the world. In the beginning I thought it was awesome to have oranges in the summer, and strawberries in the winter, but now I realize I was wrong.

So, now that you know that the food pyramid is not a "one size fits all" model, and that the quality of foods is just as important as the specific foods you eat, "What are you to do?" I recommend that you make your own food pyramid, and develop a meal plan that works for you. As you will see, at the end of this chapter, the food pyramid I created is almost reversed from the one we are familiar with. Some people are able to eat more starches or fruits, and others will have to eat less, but this is what individualizing and customizing is all about. The exact amounts and proportions will be varied according to the way your body reacts to them. You will learn the amounts and kinds of foods that you ultimately need as you accumulate more information on the way food affects you, your weight, sugar level, blood pressure, mood, and energy. You will be on your way to better health.

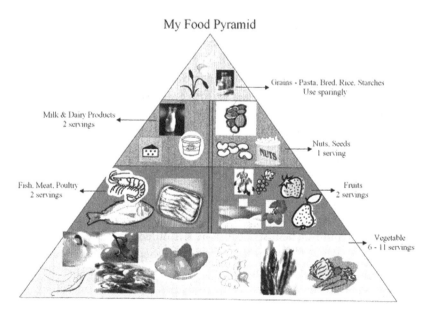

My Food Pyramid

Grains - Pasta, Bred, Rice, Starches
Use sparingly

Milk & Dairy Products
2 servings

Nuts, Seeds
1 serving

Fish, Meat, Poultry
2 servings

Fruits
2 servings

Vegetable
6 - 11 servings

———— Chapter Six ————

HABITS OLD AND NEW

Eating as a Habit

The way we eat, the type of foods we eat, and the reason we eat, are all considered to be habit-forming behaviors. I've found that our habits are either good or bad when it comes to eating. These eating habits are developed in the early years of our life. The types of foods we are exposed to and eat on a regular basis as children will become the foods that we grow most accustom to. This way we create our food memory, and the foods in our memory bank will be the ones that we crave. I believe that just as we learn to walk, speak, play, and distinguish bad from good, is also the same way we learn to like healthy foods.

I was surprised to see how many children today do not like vegetables, salads and fruits. I believe that's because they didn't learn to like them! The United States has the biggest fast food industry in the world. Growing up eating fast food, and there is one fast food place on almost every corner, is naturally what they will prefer as adults. Convenience, price, busy schedules and the fast pace of life, continues to sustain the fast food industry.

The United States has also, the highest percentage of overall obesity in the world. What's even worse is that this is among children as well. Look at their lifestyles and the types of food children eat on a regular basis, and then look at how inactive they are! Doing a random check-up to see what schools are serving for lunch, will give you an indication as to why we have such a high percentage of obese children.

In response to this obesity epidemic, big industries have come forth to produce various diet products such as food, pills and beverages. Many have us believing that we can take a simple pill to lose weight, without changing a thing about our eating habits! Well, that's deceiving because some people may lose weight temporarily, but that doesn't make them healthy. It is important that you learn more about food, so that you can change the way you think about food.

Though the word "habit" can have a negative connotation of changelessness, I do believe that improvement, or changes to food habits can be successfully made. My best proof for this was my husband's ability to effectively change his eating habits.

You must learn to eat healthy foods. Healthy eating should be a way of life, not a temporary concept of "going on a diet." How much you eat is as important as what you eat. I'll say eat to live, don't live to eat!

Doctors recommend that you eat until you feel full. This can be translated as "Eat until you no longer feel hungry." Unfortunately, the more you eat each time, the more food you will want to eat the next time. The stomach is an elastic organ that changes its size according to the amount of food you eat. The hunger sensation actually disappears shortly after you start eating. Finishing a meal is in fact an eating habit. I can still hear my mom's voice in my head "Don't get up from that table until you've finished everything on your plate." If that is the case, make sure not to put too much food on your plate in the first place. Let's say that you finish your main meal and you are still hungry. What should do you do? Instead of eating more, try adding a piece of fruit for dessert this will fill you up.

In Romania, our eating habits are different, not necessarily better, just different. Our main meal is lunch. We have a three course meal for lunch: soup, some meat with vegetables, salad, and dessert. I found that eating a salad as a side dish, instead of by itself, is more satisfying and makes it a lot easier to forget about bread. Romanians are big bread eaters and eat bread with almost every meal. Dinner on the other hand, is a lighter meal, usually consisting of a dinner salad or a sandwich. I found that in order to better control hunger, it is important to eat at the same time each day. I would say that this is imperative for diabetics, in order to keep blood sugar level and insulin at a constant level of comfortable. Healthy snacks, like raw vegetables, low-fat cheese, and fruit in between meals, will also help keep hunger and insulin under control. Therefore, you must stop making excuses such as work schedules, not enough time, and the convenience and low-cost of fast food.

Instead take a closer look at your actions, and start making the right choices for yourselves and your children.

Changing your eating habits could appear hard to do in the beginning, especially if you are the type of person that resigns changes. Taking one small step at the time will make this process successful. Start by changing one meal at a time, or by introducing one new meal at the time. Reduce the portions that you usually eat, and introduce healthy snacks like raw vegetables or fruit in between your meals. By doing this, you will be one step closer to your goal. Remember to keep making those changes, and before you know it, you will change your entire eating habits, and the way you think and feel about food.

Changing the Way We Think

Changing our eating habits and lifestyle, sounds complicated and nearly close to impossible. But, if we could only reprogram our minds the way we reprogram our computers, it would be a piece of cake–no pun intended. And, though the reality appears often difficult, it is not impossible, and the results are well worth the effort. We rely on our minds for almost everything from resisting temptations, to making decisions regarding our health, to dealing with emotions triggered by stress, anxiety, depression.

We live in a country where we have free will and the temptations of more eating options than anywhere else in the world. Making the right choices can be very hard and tricky. We have fast food restaurants at almost every corner. We have big on mouth-watering advertisements and displays, where for as much as a few pennies more, we can super-size our meal. While it is true that fast food is unhealthy, it is cheap, convenient, and right there in front of you. Moreover, it tastes good and we become addicted to it. We can't walk around blindfolded, but we can ignore them. Most importantly, *we can find better options.*

Why Do We Eat

Appetite comes in two forms: a physiological signal that makes us hungry, and emotional coaxes that lure us to food. As mentioned previously, to understand appetite, you must know that the key command center of the body is the hypothalamus gland located in the center of the brain, which controls temperature, metabolism, and sex drive. It also coordinates the behaviors that involve appetite for food and thirst. It is controlled by two counterbalancing chemicals that are located side by side. These are the satiety chemicals and eating chemicals.

For instance, fat produces a chemical signal in the brain that tells us to stop eating. The problem occurs when we override our internal monitoring system and continue to stuff ourselves long after we are no longer hungry. So the battle over eating is between our brain chemicals. It may seem that we don't have much control over the chemical reactions that take place within our bodies or inside our brain, but just as we can control cholesterol and blood pressure, by changing the foods we eat, we can also control the satiety center of the brain in the same way.

As mentioned before, my husband was big eater. I'm talking about really big portions before he would say he was no longer hungry. After the first three weeks on his diet, his portions started to reduce in size until they became reasonable. Now, his appetite is equivalent to mine. He became satisfied with less amounts of food because he was eating healthy well-balanced meals.

The same way we rely on our minds to make the right choices, we rely on our tongue to relay information about food. The information we acquire sends messages to the brain, and the brain sends messages back, this tells us to continue or to stop eating. The messages come largely from our tastes recognition of sweet, sour, salty, and bitter, as well as from what we smell. According to scientists, 75% of the taste of certain foods actually comes from how we smell it. The physiological makeup of our tongue could make us more or less disposed to eating good or bad foods.

How Do We Change?

Early in life we develop eating habits. Our family, culture, and lifestyle play a decisive role in formulating our eating habits. We also create and develop food memory, which is why we usually crave something that is starchy, sugary, or loaded with fat, because we *remember* that it tastes good. One big step on our path to reprogramming our mind will be to first change and rebuild the images in our food memory, and by learning to enjoy good healthy foods. I've found healthy recipes come in handy.

If possible, find good recipes that make appealing presentations on your plate. Also, when you take the first bite, hold it in your mouth a little bit, savor the aroma, and then tell yourself how good that tastes. Do that consistently every time, and you will change the way you remember and think about food.

I agree that it is hard to break bad habits. I deal with this realization every day at our gymnastic facility. I've found it helpful that when considering the development of new habits, concentrate on effective making new ones, and not on breaking old ones. Making changes in our lives is as much mental as it is behavioral. Think about the behavior that you're seeking to establish, then decide in your mind that *you* want to succeed, and are ready to make that change. Then start creating new habits that will support *your* goal.

We talk about improving the quality of many facets of our lives, including our education, jobs, homes, schools for our children, relationships, neighborhoods, and even more mundane things like our cars and clothing, and yet we somehow pay less attention to our health or the foods we eat. I suppose the reason for this is that we are too busy with other things.

Think about it. When we decide we want a better job, a new car, or house, we do everything we can in our power to get it. We plan, budget and work harder. But, when it comes to food, somehow we seem to fail. It seems to be such a daunting task to change how we eat, whether we're diabetic or simply trying to lose weight, and control our cholesterol and blood pressure. Why is this?

Food is tied into so much of what we do on a day to day basis. It's the highlight of celebrations, and at the center of social gatherings. Like a good friend, food is reliable and dependable—always there when you need it. For as long as there have been communities, food and love have been celebrated and associated in one way or another. For example, we eat turkey for Thanksgiving, lamb for Easter, and pork for Christmas (at least in my tradition). Food is a must have due to tradition, which is also linked to food memory. The same goes for how we think about desserts. We associate certain desserts with certain occasions.

Moreover, some of us are emotional eaters. Therefore, on those non-occasions when faced with day to day challenges, we usually turn to food for comfort, especially desserts. We often respond to the traumas or realities that have caused unpleasant feelings by eating our way out. The reality is that in order to truly enjoy the things we desire—the material possessions, improved relationships, or true happiness—we must first seek to improve our health, with as much zeal as pursuing that new car, job, or house. We cannot fully enjoy the things of life, until we are healthy.

You have to make lifestyle changes, in order to affect your blood sugar level, blood pressure, weight, or overall health. You must make up your mind to change the way you see things before you can change your eating habits. Food should be only one of the things to enjoy in life, and not the centerpiece. The incentive to change should come from deep within you. In order to change your live, you should change the way you think, because the way you think determines the way you feel, in turn influencing the way you act.

My husband also had to change the way he thought about food, particularly about his diet. He was growing tired of depriving himself of the foods he liked due to him trying so many diets, especially while getting no results. Just the word "deprive" makes you feel frustrated, angry, and against the whole idea of "going on a diet." This is why I kept the majority of my recipes more or less the same. I changed the ingredients to make them healthier. We also maintained an "indulging" day, and kept our holiday food traditions intact. These days were exceptions, but not the rule for how we ate on a regular basis.

What Can We Change?

Shortly after I began my research, I understood that we were approaching the whole concept of "dieting" from a rather shortsighted view. We are doomed to fail if we approach diets with the mentality that it is a temporary deprivation or "fix," and as soon as we have achieved our goal, we can return to our old eating habits. A diet should be a common manner of living. A diet is simply a regimen of changes in the areas of behavior and attitudes about food and exercise.

How do we know what to change? Where do we begin?

First, everyone should learn more about nutrition and the effect of specific foods on their body. Keep records of the foods *you* eat, and how *your* body reacts to them. Included in this your sugar level and how foods make you feel in the long run. We are all different and therefore, it is important to know and understand the many factors that make us metabolically and bio-chemically different.

Find out which foods disagree with you, which ones give you energy, and those that make you tired or bloated. Become familiar with how specific foods alter your mood, and learn what proportions of carbohydrate, fat, and protein are right for you. Knowing this information will help you design your own meal plan, and create your own goals and strategies to help you achieve a healthier lifestyle.

As mentioned, my husband tried all kinds of diets, including many of those on the market, as well as those prescribed by dieticians. Unfortunately, none of these helped him significantly lower his blood sugar level or lose the fat around his midsection. Those diets weren't necessarily bad diets; they just were not right *for him*. Our major goal in finding the right diet for my husband was to bring his sugar levels under control. In a diet, diabetics require foods that produce a balanced hormonal response. High circulating levels of insulin have to be limited, due to the fact in its presence, fat cannot be burned adequately. A diet that recommends six to eleven servings of grains such as bread, pasta or cereal, will not only fatten you, but in my husband's case, caused diabetic conditions. I discovered that insulin is primarily triggered by large meals, carbohydrates, and to a lesser degree by protein.

Everyone especially diabetics, needs foods that will slowly raise the blood sugar to a comfortable level, and maintain that level for a long time. Believe me, being a diabetic, and self-employed, make it difficult to acquire health insurance. As a result, visits to the doctors and nutritionists, along with lab tests can become very costly. This is why it is so important to learn about your body and understand how your body responds to different foods and diets. We are all different, therefore, we will respond differently.

The only way that my husband and I succeeded in our efforts to make lifestyle changes was by learning everything we could about food, body functions, and the effect of specific foods that we monitored closely. We made a food diary, in which we recorded when, and what types of food my husband ate. We also recorded the effects of the foods that were eaten, including sugar level, moods, hunger sensations, and his personal reactions to different foods. I recommend this approach to everyone, as it allows you to do your own self-observation, and make the necessary adjustments. This is the only way that you can ever understand what works for *you, and only you!*

It Is Not Easy but It Can Be Done

Finding and maintaining the right diet is definitely not easy. It takes time and willpower to make changes in our lives, create new habits, and learn to like new foods. At the beginning of your new diet, you will have to exercise more control and not give in to cravings. As a result, over time you will learn how to eat right and manage your cravings. Eating right will become automatic, as you will have established new habits to help you. It is also very important to set realistic goals for yourself, and develop ways to achieve them. Be patient. Do not expect to drop several pounds in a short amount of time. Don't expect your sugar level to drop on the very first day that you start eating healthy. Give your body time to reset itself.

When we started this new self-discovery diet, my husband was very skeptical and impatient. After all, we had tried everything we were told, and nothing worked. He no longer believed that anything would work. He wanted proof, and he wanted it quick! I would ask him, "What do you have to lose?" In other words, if we fail to succeed, we come out of it with a new experience, having lost nothing. But if we do succeed, think about how wonderful it will be, to be freed from diabetes!"

Even so, changing our eating behaviors takes responsibility, commitment, and inner strength; it also helps to have support. What support is better than the support that comes from your family? This is why I use the collective pronoun "we." We were in this together, despite the fact that I myself am not a diabetic, nor do I have cholesterol or blood pressure problems. I just believe that it's important to learn to eat and live healthy, in order to ensure the quality of life that we have together. Having the right support is critical in our efforts to adopt healthier lifestyles.

Imagine how difficult it would be to suddenly start eating broccoli, when the person that sits across from you is eating a juicy steak and fries! It's like a smoker that continues to smoke, but tells you all the reasons that *you* should stop smoking. I am familiar with the saying "Do as I say, and not as I do" but that doesn't help with personal motivation. One of the things that I often tell my gymnasts, is that motivation means desire, and we must remember to hold on to it, when it competes with other desires. In their case, they would rather hang out with friends or watch movies, instead of being in the gym training hard. In your case you have to overcome the tiredness after the workouts, and the cravings for deserts or salty snacks.

How? By staying motivated and not giving in. It is easier to stay motivated along the way if you have a big picture in front of you. In my gymnasts' case, the ultimate goal is to go to the Olympics, or get a college scholarship. In my husband's case, it is to manage and build a better life with diabetes. You have to design a path, take small steps, set realistic goals, and seek to achieve them one at the time. If you do this, you will get there. Motivation is all about making the right choice during tempting situations. Each meal, and exercise session is a decision, which puts you further from your goal or closer to it. In our case, I applied the same advice that I gave my gymnasts every day; practice is the key to success! Practicing healthy eating and consistent exercising will create and develop new healthy habits that will ultimately help you enhance the quality of your life. Living with diabetes, losing weight, and lowering blood pressure and cholesterol is not easy. It takes time but face it, so does everything else that's worth it.

One of the things, I've wonder about is, "Why do most diets fail?" One of the reasons is that we tend to lose our motivation. We expect quick results, since almost all diets present us with the deceptive picture, claiming that we will loose the weight "fast." Needless to say, when that doesn't work, we quit!

Staying Motivated Is the Key to Success

We can stay motivated by setting small goals, achieving them one at a time, and being very proud of our achievements. The most important thing is to never say "*I can't.*" We can do whatever we set our minds to. In our gym, I see obese kids on a daily basis who become easily discouraged when learning to tumble. They have a harder time since they have the extra weight to carry, and want to give up after their first try. I always tell them that they can accomplish and master this skill if they take it one step at the time. I also tell them to be patient, and continue training. The same applies to managing and overcoming diabetes, high cholesterol, high blood pressure, or any other metabolic disorder. Knowing your body and its functions, and how foods affect your body, along with implementing necessary changes, will ensure that you accomplish your goals. As result, you *will* get your blood sugar under control; improve your health, and the quality of your life. You will be a winner!

Success from a particular diet will vary from one person to the next, because we each have a unique metabolism. Embracing ourselves is an important part of accepting our limitations, and making the proper adjustments to maintain over the long term. Having the information that you need about how your body works will further equip you to make those changes. Lifestyle reprogramming and eating reeducation are both difficult things to do, but as I told my husband, your body does not care how difficult it is, it only deals with the end results. This is why it is important to really look at what's in your diet, not only the calories, but also the amount of carbohydrate, fat, and protein that it contains on a daily basis. This will prevent you from assuming that something is healthy when in fact, it is not.

As you become more educated about nutrition, you will be more likely to buy and consume foods that are healthy. For example, when possible, buy lean meats that are antibiotic and steroids free. Also reduce, if not eliminate your intake of pesticides and chemical additives, by buying organic foods. The focus should be on the quality of your diet. All foods are not created equally; therefore we need more of some than others.

Once you've learned which foods are healthy for you, take inventory of the foods in your kitchen pantry and begin eliminating the unhealthy ones. Learn to listen to your body and eat for the right reasons. Restructure the way you think about food and eating. In addition, make sure to incorporate exercise into your daily schedule. Change your attitude, be positive and open minded about trying new foods and food preparations. Make sure to practice good habits and behavior towards food and you will change your life. Remember, there are far greater things to do in life than living to eat! **I say, "Eat to live!"**

Chapter Seven

EXERCISE
A MUST OR A HOBBY?

Life today is very fast paced. We are always busy on the run, or otherwise trying to achieve a balance between work and family. The list goes on and on, and it seems that we don't even have time to stop and catch our breath, much less think about ourselves and what we truly need.

Technological advances and modern conveniences have made our lives safer, more comfortable, and less complicated, yet we are more stressed and have even less time for life's most important things, such as taking care of ourselves and incorporating regular physical activity into our lives. Just think about how much simpler life has become. For instance, our electronic garage door openers allow us to remain in our cars, and with the touch of a button, we can simply pull into our garages. Riding lawn mowers enable us to cut the grass without moving a muscle, and light vacuum cleaners allow us to do hardly any lifting. The abundance of precooked meals that proliferate the supermarket shelves, and the prevalence of fast food restaurants make it easier for us to cook less, and help feed the notion that we need these conveniences to sustain the fast pace of our lives and ultimately save us more time. What big time savers!

But my question is, "Who actually has the time to consider the true price that we pay for all the convenience in terms of our health?" I don't remember growing up and seeing so many obese children and adults, and there certainly weren't as many cases of diabetes. But life was different back then. Children played outside more, and were more physically active. In fact they did not sit on the sofa all day and play video games. Instead, they were an active part of the games. Back then, parents had more time to prepare home-cooked meals, and take walks in the park in the evening with the family. Many times, they even walked to the grocery store. Though there were fewer "conveniences," including fast food places and time-saving technologies, we had more time, and as a result, we were also less stressed. The bottom line is that we ate healthier and were more physically active.

Today, not only has our way of living changed, but food has changed as well. We see such changes as from the way they are grown to the way they are manufactured. They have become less natural, with higher contents of hormones, antibiotics and pesticides. In spite of all these changes, you still have the ability to make better and informed choices. Knowing and understanding the contribution of foods and your body and its functions will enable you to make smart decisions about how and what you eat.

But, what about exercise? This is an equally important part of the formula for a healthy life and body. I consider exercise a *must*. Human activity centers around the capability to provide energy on a continuous basis. Without a continuous source of energy, cells and muscles cease to function and die. Energy is provided through the metabolic breakdown of two principal sources: carbohydrates and fats. Amino acids are the building blocks of proteins and provide a small quantity of energy during exercise. Both exercise and physical activity helps us to increase our energy expenditure. However, there is a difference between the two of them.

We all participate in some type of physical activity, from making the bed, cleaning the house and preparing food, to more continuous activities such as running, biking, or swimming. Though we are "active" when doing routine activities of daily living, the energy expenditure differs greatly versus when we perform exercise, where energy is provided on a more long-term, or continuous basis.

Exercise is usually performed during leisure time with the specific intention of improving one's physical fitness. But, because it is performed during leisure "downtime," we usually find excuses to not do it. My husband and I are guilty of this when we use excuses such as: "I don't have time," or "I am too tired," or "I am active enough at work." Or, perhaps the most commonly used one, "I will start tomorrow." Once you become familiar with the benefits of regular exercise, and begin to see and feel the results, you will want to make a hobby out of it. No one has an abundance of leisure time, but somehow we seem to find the time to do what we consider to be important to us.

Just as with food, we must also approach exercise similarly, from the perspective of habit formation. It is about changing behavior, and integrating these new behaviors as habits in our daily lives. When it comes to incorporating exercise into our daily lives, many people ultimately quit because they place too much of an emphasis on the amount of exercise that they do and how quickly it will produce results. This is a reflection of our impatience.

Our life runs at a fast pace, and we want quick results. When my gymnasts first join the competitive team, both they and their parents all want to know how long it will take them before they are ready to compete. I tell them to be patient. There is a progression of skills development that they must follow and achieve in order to become competitive. The time will vary based on the individual. Skill building has to start slowly, while taking into consideration injury prevention, and more importantly, individual fitness levels.

Given this knowledge, you should keep in mind that how much you do all at once is not as important as doing something consistently over time. This is how you successfully develop and maintain new habits. You should never compare yourself, the type of exercise you do, the duration or your endurance level with anybody else. Always measure your success based on your own progress. This is the only way that you will enjoy exercise, and then and only then will you incorporate it in your daily routine.

According to the American Heart Association (2008, U.S. American Heart Association) there are four risk factors for coronary heart disease. These are referred to as the "the major modifiable risk factors": physical inactivity, smoking, high blood pressure and elevated total blood cholesterol level. Although there are other risk factors for having a heart attack such as age, heredity, diabetes, gender, and stress, the big four are linked to lifestyle choices. This is why it is critical that exercise becomes a priority and part of your life routine. It can be the best choice that anybody can make.

Benefits of Exercise: "The Magnificent Thirteen"

I learned that Type 2 Diabetes is caused by resistance of peripheral tissues (skeletal muscles) to insulin which stimulates glucose uptake. Exercise in conjunction with diet and/or drug therapy improves glycemic control (blood sugar level), reduces certain cardiovascular risk factors, and enhances psychological well being. This is why exercise is critical for a diabetic person. Exercise has many benefits, but I chose the ones that I consider to be most important. I like to call these the "magnificent thirteen."

1. Regular exercise improves cell membrane insulin sensitivity,

glucose transport across the cell membrane, and lowers insulin plasma levels.

2. HDL cholesterol can be beneficially influenced by constant aerobic exercise. Triglycerides represent a fuel source for skeletal muscles, and elevated volumes can be reduced if exercise series are repeated on regular basis. Remember the huge drop in my husband's triglycerides level after just one month of diet and exercise. Unless the exercise regimen is associated with the loss of body fat or improved dietary habits, exercise by itself does not lower total body cholesterol or LDL.

3. We all know that with advancing age, it is normal for a person to become out of shape, lose muscular strength and flexibility, and experience an increase in blood pressure, body weight and cholesterol. The truth is that there is a clear decrease in cardiorespiratory fitness with age. Skeletal muscles are affected; there is a reduction of muscle size, strength, and capillarization. Muscles serve as a primary energy consumer for the body. If we are inactive, we lose an average of 5% of our muscle mass every ten years after the age of 35. As our muscles age, we lose some of the proteins that make up the muscles; these are what give the muscles the ability to have both strength and stamina. Exercise training however, has been shown to reverse these changes. Resistance training, specifically, has been shown to increase the protein synthesis of muscles.

4. Exercise decreases insulin levels by enhancing the glucose uptake by muscles. It appears that a small amount of insulin is adequate and necessary to permit these exercise-related increases in glucose uptake. This increase in insulin sensitivity, where less or the same amount of insulin is able to do the job, is present for at least 48 hours after just one hour of moderate exercise.

5. Exercise helps to reduce fat. To break down fat, we first have to use up glycogen, which can take up to a half hour of exercise. That is when the body automatically begins to burn fat. Exercise keeps total body fat content low and may reduce the rate at which adipose cells accumulate.

6. Exercise helps you to lose the extra weight. If a given

food intake does not allow weight reduction, the physical activity must be increased for a negative energy balance to occur. Activities must be selected that require long-term energy expenditure, but at the same time be within the limits of your own physical and skill capabilities. Exercise rebuilds and maintains proteins and muscle mass to prevent us from gaining weight.

7. Exercise keeps the blood vessels open and clog-free. The blood functions better when it is fluid rather then viscous, which means flowing easily through the capillaries. Exercise, by keeping the blood fluid, could help prevent a stroke or a heart attack. One measure of the fluidity of the blood is the "stickiness" of the platelets—particles that are important for the normal formation of a blood clot after a cut—but they can do harm if they precipitate a clot in the blood vessel, since such a clot can block one of the large vessels that goes to the brain or to the heart, causing a stroke or a heart attack.

8. Exercise increases metabolism, so we burn more energy at a higher rate. It also helps reduce the appetite by turning on the sympathetic nervous system, helping burn more calories, thus losing weight.

9. Exercise reduces stress. We all experience stress, and reducing it in any way we can is very important. Under stress, the production of adrenaline is increased, which causes fat cells to release fat into the blood stream to be used as energy. In response, the adrenal glands produce too much cortisol (the stress hormone) to handle the fat in the blood stream. This stress hormone is known to cause fat storage in the abdominal area. High cortisol levels reduce insulin sensitivity. The kidney responds to high cortisol levels by retaining salt and water, which increases the blood pressure.

10. Exercise helps decrease depression and increase a positive attitude. The beneficial effect of exercise on our psyche results from elevation of certain hormones called beta-endorphin, which are very potent mood elevators. This is why we feel better and more energized after we exercise. Our thinking is usually clearer and our overall mood is elevated. I don't know about you, but when I am physically

active, whether in the kitchen or cleaning the house, or walking on the treadmill, I am always able to clear my mind, and solve my daily problems.

11. Exercise builds a stronger heart, and a stronger heart is a healthier heart! A strong heart works more efficiently; delivering more blood per beat, thereby requiring fewer beats to pump the same amount of blood. Each stroke is stronger, and the amount of blood delivered with each stroke is increased with exercise training. Also, like the rest of the body, the heart muscles improve their ability to extract oxygen from blood with exercise training. This is very important in the case where one may have blockages that have reduced the amount of the blood flow, for the heart can extract more oxygen from less blood.

12. Exercise builds collateral vessels. When arteries to the heart muscles start to fill with fatty deposits, the body's normal defense is to build additional blood vessels around the artery to ensure continued blood flow. I read that many times a heart artery will close completely, but a heart attack is avoided because collateral arteries have developed around the blockage. It has been proven that regular exercise help to distance us from the disease, atherosclerosis. Also, we can speed up the development of collateral circulation by exercising, and according to the scientists, exercise is the only activity that can achieve this.

13. Exercise helps to lower blood pressure. Although the treatment of hypertension involves the use of medication designed to decrease plasma volume (diuretics), regular and moderate exercise, has been shown to lead to a sustained decrease in both systolic and diastolic pressure. Assessed over time, exercise training may lower blood pressure to the point that less medication or no medication might be needed. My husband was able to lower his medication dosage after two months of diet and exercise, and was free of medication after five months.

How to Get Started

There are various reasons for not exercising. Some are physiological, behavioral and psycho-social. They can also include a lack of time, personal safety, social environment, medical problems, self image, self discipline, or a lack of knowledge. Current estimates are that 20% to 60% of people who started an exercise program eventually stop (U.S. Department of Health and Human Services, 2007). There are various reasons for stopping such as smoking, enjoyment, injury, timing, age, gender, level of education. I believe the main reason we stop exercising is due to the way we think about exercise in the first place. It is also the same reason why many diets fail, and many people continuously go on and off diets. Apart from the fact that some diets really don't work, or are too strict or complicated, most of us tend to approach diets and exercise as temporary phases.

We all tend to set our goal, whether it's to lose ten or twenty pounds, and we "go on a diet." But the question is, "Then what?" What do we do once we've lost the weight? Often times it is common for us, to revert back to our bad eating habits that got us in trouble in the first place. Moreover, if we don't lose the desired amount of pounds in a short time, we quit! Conversely, if we changed our thinking about diet and exercise, and approached it more as a lifestyle change and better way to live, we would be more successful. In turn, we would be more convinced of the merits of such an approach, and ultimately change the way we live our lives.

At first, my husband didn't believe in the significance or benefits of exercise. He just wasn't willing to give up the little bit of leisure time that he had. On one hand, I understood he was already active in the gym, and our work schedule did not leave us with a lot of downtime. But, I told him to think of exercise much like the medication he was taking for his diabetes on a regular basis. I was not surprised that what initially started as a duty soon became part of his daily routine.

If you are not currently an active person, start your exercise program slowly, according to your fitness level and limitations dictated by your medical condition. Choose light exercise for shorter periods of time and gradually increase the intensity and duration. A little physical activity goes a long way. Even in the busiest of lives today, any one can combine a series of shorter duration activities such as climbing the stairs instead of taking the elevator, and walking during the day. The point is to be as active as you can, as part of your everyday life.

How Much Physical Activity Do I Need?

According to ACSM (American College of Sports Medicine, 2007, Statement on exercise), all children and adults should accumulate a minimum of 30 minutes, performed in bouts of 10 minutes or more, of moderate and/or vigorous physical activity, on most and preferably all days of the week. When choosing an exercise regimen, there are factors that should be taken in consideration, such as effectiveness, safety, optimal dose of exercise, minimized injuries, and achievable benefit expected.

Accumulated physical activity means that it does not matter how calories are expended over the course of a day, as long as they are expended at a moderate to high intensity, to achieve the desired effect. Get involved in some kind of exercise at least three times a week. Some good examples of exercise are aerobics, playing basketball, dancing, or just walking during sometime of the day. Increase leisure activities and reduce periods of inactivity times in any possible way.

Muscles

Knowing your muscles is as important as knowing your body functions and your foods.

Skeletal muscles are the muscles attached to the bones by tendons and ligaments, and they come in pairs. They are designed to do two things: make us fast and make us strong. While muscles give us the metabolic ability to burn calories every time we move, their true advantage is that they constantly feed on calories. Every pound of muscle burns between 40-120 calories/day, just to sustain itself, while every pound of fat feeds on 1-3 calories/day. By focusing on the right muscles and following the right plan, you will be able to firm up without adding bulk. We all would like to have firm, nice looking bodies, rather than cellulite, and it's possible without major effort. Though it isn't as easy or quick as taking a pill, we can achieve many health benefits, not to mention improved appearance, just by becoming active.

There are two main forms of exercise: stamina training and strength training. These influence the structure of the muscles differently. **Stamina training** increases the muscles' capacity to produce and use energy they need to contract. While **strength training** makes a bigger, stronger, and sturdier muscle fiber structure. By strength training on a regular basis, we create more muscle mass.

Muscles serve as primary energy consumers for the body. As I mentioned, as muscles age, we lose some of the proteins that make up the muscles; they are what give the muscles the ability to have both strength and stamina. Exercise rebuilds and maintains proteins and muscle mass to prevent us from gaining weight.

The type of exercise that I would say is critical for a diabetic person, and it is the one with which my husband started, is low in intensity, but high in compliance. A good example of this would be walking, which enhances the reduction of body fat and minimizes injuries. Frequency of exercise can range from four to seven days a week, for duration of 20 to 60 minutes, in accordance to your fitness level, age and your medical condition.

My husband started his exercise regimen with walking every morning for 20 minutes, and then he increased his time to 30 minutes after a one-week period. After two weeks, he started walking in the morning *and* evening for 30 minutes at a time. After the third week, he added strength training every other day for 20 minutes at a time. Today, he continues to follow the same exercise regimen, except that now he includes strength training as a daily component for 30 minutes. He feels great and he is in great shape. We laugh sometimes, when we recall how difficult it was when he first started walking in the morning, in comparison to how easy everything feels now.

Types of Exercise

A. Walking

You can be creative when walking, whether you do it around the house, from the farther parking lot space to the store door, at work or outside, or on the treadmill, just make sure that you walk for an accumulated 30 minutes a day. If you can also join a fitness club, but I personally found the membership fees to be somewhat expensive and inconvenient. Therefore, my husband and I decided to buy a treadmill. This way we could walk in the morning, hop in the shower and get ready for work, all in the same amount of time that it would have taking us to drive back and forth to the fitness club. Always use walking as a warm-up before you start your exercise regimen. Once you are warmed up, you can start with 10 minutes of fast walking, followed by 20 minutes of strength training, and 5 minutes of stretch time.

B. Strength Training

Strength training helps rebuild the muscle fibers and increases muscle mass, so that you can burn calories more efficiently. Train the big muscles that make up the core axis of the body such as legs, chest, shoulders, back and the abdominal. You can do this at the fitness club, or follow the exercises that my husband and I are doing. You can strength train by using your body's weight or by using dumbbells, rubber tubing, or ankle weights. You can purchase these at almost any sports store or retailer with a sports section. They are rather inexpensive and useful.

Note of caution: If you use rubber tubing make sure that you stretch and relax the tubing in a very smoothly controlled fashion. Do not let the tubing "snap" quickly back after it is stretched, because this motion may cause injury.

Divide your strength training exercise into two phases. The length of the first phase should be determined by your fitness level and age. If you are a beginner, I would recommend anywhere between 12 to 16 weeks. The intensity of the exercise should be kept low, but with high volume. The purpose of this phase is to gradually prepare the muscles and their tendon attachments to the bones for the more intense training that follows in phase two, where the intensity steadily increases while volume gradually decreases. The times to switch from phase one to phase two will be dictated by your body. When you feel that you perform your exercises easily, with no effort and they no longer fatigue your muscles, it is time to challenge yourself and move on to phase two.

Exercises are divided into 9 groups according to the group of muscles being worked. They are listed in order of intensity, beginning from low to high intensity. Choose one exercise from each group each week, starting with the first one. Allow yourself to train in a circuit fashion. I have included the recommended number of repetitions and weeks for each exercise within each group. I also recommend that the exercises be performed in this order to allow for proper rest between sets. The effectiveness of the exercise is compromised without proper rest in between sets. When training to improve power, it is important to allow at least 3-6 minutes of rest before stimulating the same muscle group. It is possible to gain strength and power without creating unnecessary muscle hypertrophy. This is especially important for women, as hypertrophy of muscles can create added weight or bulky muscles. Start by rotating through the training circuit one time, then increase to two, ultimately achieving three rotations per strength training session.

Remember you should start your strength training by performing it every other day. It takes a day of rest in between strength training sessions for a fully fatigued muscle to recover. If adequate time for the muscle to recuperate and adapt to the training stimulus is not allowed, then progressive muscle breakdown may occur, resulting in decreased strength and increased risk of injuries.

Group I: Legs

The quadriceps muscle is primarily strengthened in the exercises.

1. Lateral steps-ups

Stand with your feet on an object (for instance, a block, aerobic step, stool or a set of stairs). The height of the object should be low enough so that the knee will not bend greater than 90 degrees. Slowly lower the opposite foot down to the floor, keeping the foot flexed so that only the heel touches, then return to starting position. Perform three sets per side.

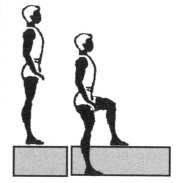

Week 1: 10 Reps
Week 2: 12 Reps
Week 3: 15 Reps

2. Front lunges

Stand with your feet shoulder width apart, hands on your hips. Take a long step forward with your left foot; bend your left knee making sure that it does not extend pass your toes, keeping body weight on both legs to assure that your back is straight. Pause, then step back to the original standing position. Repeat, by stepping forward with your right foot. Perform two sets per side.

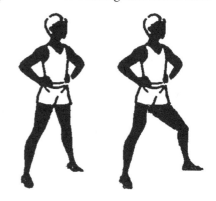

Week 4: 12 Reps
Week 5: 14 Reps
Week 6: 16 Reps

3. Squats

Stand with your feet shoulder width apart, arms at your side. Without arching your back, slowly bend your knees until your thighs are almost parallel to the ground; inhale on your way down. As you bend, bring your arms straight in front of you at shoulder height for balance. Pause while squeezing your thighs and glutes. Return to the original standing position, with your arms at side; exhale on your way up. Perform two sets.

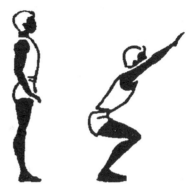

Week 7: 12 Reps
Week 8: 15 Reps
Week 9: 18 Reps

4. Leg extensions

Sit on a sturdy chair with your back straight against the back of chair, wearing ankle weights. Slowly extend your legs in front of you. Pause; then slowly return your legs to the initial position. Perform one set.

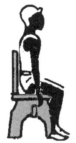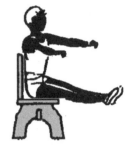

Week 10: 10 Reps
Week 11: 12 Reps
Week 12: 14 Reps

5. One leg squat in lunge position

Facing forward, while standing, lift your left leg backwards and upwards, to place your left foot on a chair, sofa, or other leveled surface, with your heel facing up. Slowly bend the right knee until your thigh is nearly parallel to the ground. In this lunge position, your knee should not pass your toes. Do not lunge below the level of the sofa or chair. Slowly straighten your leg to return to the original position. Repeat the exercise with the other leg. Perform one set.

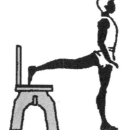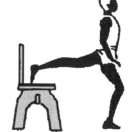

Week 13: 12 Reps
Week 14: 14 Reps
Week 15: 14 Reps

Group II: Chest/Arms/Triceps

As the name implies, this group primarily stimulates the triceps, chest, and shoulders. It is very important to control the trunk when performing these exercises. You can do this by squeezing the buttocks and contracting the lower abdominal muscles. This will improve the strength of your core and help reduce back injuries.

1. Push-ups

Get in a standard push-up position with your hands shoulder width apart. Bend at the elbows while maintaining a tight trunk, until your chin almost touches the floor; then push back up. Inhale on your way down, exhale on your way up.

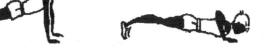

Week 1: 15 Reps
Week 2: 20 Reps
Week 3: 25 Reps

If you are a beginner and you cannot do a push-up yet, start with push-ups against the wall. Stand in front of a wall; place your hands on the wall, shoulder width apart, with your arms straight, keeping the same tight trunk. Bend arms at the elbows until your chin almost touches the wall; then push back up. Perform the same number of reps.

2. Pull-ups

Stand with your feet shoulder width apart, holding one dumbbell in each hand with thumbs pointed to each other. Keeping your arms and back straight, lift your arms up until your hands are above your shoulder; then return to the starting position. Quickly raise arms while inhaling, then slowly lower arms while exhaling.

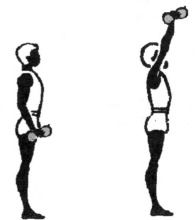

Week 4: 15 Reps
Week 5: 17 Reps
Week 6: 19 Reps

3. Elevated feet push-ups

Get in a standard push-up position with your hands shoulder width apart and your feet on a block or a low chair with a sturdy support. Bend at the elbows while maintaining a tight core, until your chin almost touches the floor; then push back up. Inhale on your way down, exhale on your way up.

Week 7: 15 Reps
Week 8: 18 Reps
Week 9: 20 Reps

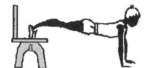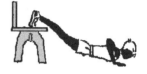

4. Lateral pull backs

While lying face down on the floor, hold one dumbbell in each hand, palms facing up. Keeping your arms straight, pull the dumbbells up just past your buttocks, hold, then return to the starting position. Maintain your back straight making sure not to arch it.

Week 10: 10 Reps
Week 11: 12 Reps
Week 12: 14 Reps

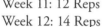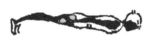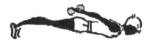

5. Triceps kickback

Place left knee on a sturdy chair, while standing, using left hand for stability. Hold a dumbbell in your right hand, while keeping your back flat, and bend your elbow to about a 90 degree angle, raising it to just about the level of your back. This is the starting position. Extend your forearm backward, keeping your upper arm stationary. When fully extended, your arm should be parallel to the ground. Pause; then return to the starting position. Repeat 20 times then switch to left arm.

Week 13: 20 Reps
Week 14: 25 Reps
Week 15: 30 Reps

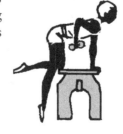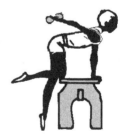

Group III: Buttocks/Hamstrings/Hips

This group is an extremely important part of any work-out and conditioning program. While we use our quadriceps frequently during daily activities, we tend to neglect our hamstrings, which are situated directly behind our quadriceps. In order to prevent a significant muscular imbalance between these two muscle groups, the hamstrings must be incorporated into any workout program, and the best exercise for this muscle is the hamstring curl. In addition to the hamstrings, this group also includes the hip abductors, the groin (hip adductors), and the buttocks.

1. Hamstring curls

Using ankle weights lie face down. Try not to arch your back throughout the exercise. A pad (mat or towel) may be placed underneath the waist. "Curl" your legs over the hamstring muscle unto the buttocks, by slowly raising your feet toward your buttocks, and slowly return to the starting position.

Week 1: 10 Reps
Week 2: 12 Reps
Week 3: 15 Reps

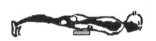 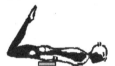

2. Straddle-n-close

Using ankle weights lie with your back flat on the floor, making sure not to arch your lower back. Lift both legs straight up together to a vertical position with your feet towards the ceiling, keeping your butt on the floor. This is the starting position. Slowly open your legs out to the side into a straddle position, with your legs as close to the floor as comfortable. Slowly bring your legs back together to return to the starting position.

Week 4: 10 Reps
Week 5: 12 Reps
Week 6: 15 Reps

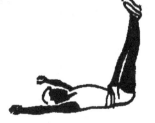 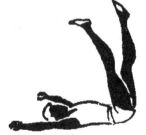

3. Back scissor

Using ankle weights lie face down on the floor, with your head resting on a towel and your arms next to your head. Keeping your legs straight, lift your feet five inches off the floor and move them up and down in a scissor-like motion.

Week 7: 15 Reps
Week 8: 18 Reps
Week 9: 20 Reps

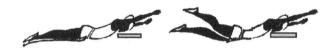

4. Hip abduction

Using ankle weights, lie on the floor on your left side. Tighten left quadriceps muscle, and in a slow and controlled motion, lift top leg 8-10 inches away from floor. Keep your legs fully extended with your feet flexed. Perform recommended number of repetitions; then repeat on the other side.

Week 10: 10 Reps
Week 11: 15 Reps
Week 12: 18 Reps

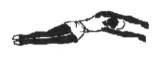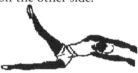

5. Hip adduction

Using ankle weights, lie on the floor on the right side of your body. Bend the upper leg and cross it over the bottom leg with the foot resting on the floor. Tighten muscle on front of thigh; then in a slow and controlled movement, lift the bottom leg 8-10 inches away from the floor. Perform the recommended number of reps; then repeat on the other side.

Week 13: 10 Reps
Week 14: 15 Reps
Week 15: 18 Reps

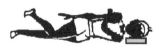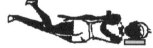

Group IV: Arms

1. Front lifts

Stand with one dumbbell in each hand, palms facing down in front of you. Maintain your alignment, by keeping your spine neutral and contracting abdomen and buttocks. Slowly lift your arms up until your hands are just above your forehead. Slowly lower your arms to return to the starting position.

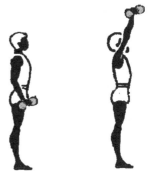

Week 1: 10 Reps
Week 2: 12 Reps
Week 3: 15 Reps

2. Kip Pull

Lie on your back on the floor with your knees bent to protect your back. Hold one dumbbell in each hand and rest your arms on the floor above your head, with palm facing up. Lift your arms in one quick motion until your hands are just above your stomach; then slowly lower your arms to return to the starting position.

Week 4: 10 Reps
Week 5: 12 Reps
Week 6: 15 Reps

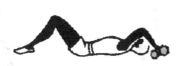 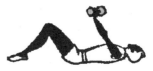

3. Partial Lateral Lifts

Stand with one dumbbell in each hand, arms at your sides, palms facing inward. Maintain your alignment by keeping your spine neutral, contracting your abdomen and buttocks. Slowly lift your arms up away from your sides, until your arms are at shoulder level; hold, then lower your arms to return to the starting position.

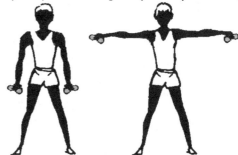

Week 7: 10 Reps
Week 8: 12 Reps
Week 9: 15 Reps

4. Complete Lateral Lifts

Stand with one dumbbell in each hand, arms at your sides, palms facing inward.

Maintain your alignment by keeping your spine neutral, contracting your abdomen and buttocks. Lift your arms until they are straight up above your shoulders. Slowly lower your arms to return to the starting position.

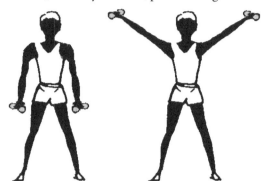

Week 10: 10 Reps
Week 11: 12 Reps
Week 12: 15 Reps

5. Reverse Lateral Lifts

Stand with one dumbbell in each hand, arms at sides, palms facing forward.

Maintain your alignment by keeping your spine neutral, contracting your abdomen and buttocks. Slowly lift your arms away from your sides until your hands are at the shoulder level; hold, then lower your arms to return to the starting position.

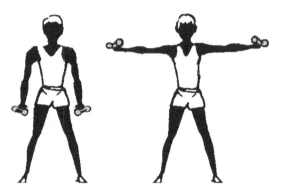

Week 13: 10 Reps
Week 14: 12 Reps
Week 15: 15 Reps

Group V: Lower leg/ calf

1. Calf Raises

Stand straight with your feet slightly apart. Lift your weight on to the balls of your feet until you feel a full stretch in your ankles, keeping your buttocks and your abs tight. Hold; then return slowly to the starting position.

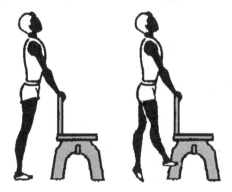

Week 1: 20 Reps
Week 2: 25 Reps
Week 3: 30 Reps

2. Single Leg Calf Raises

Stand straight with your feet slightly apart, with a sturdy chair in front of you for support. Place one hand on the back of the chair for support. Lift your weight on to the ball of the foot closest to the chair, slightly elevating the other leg in front. Rise up fast, and return slowly to the starting position. Perform the recommended number of reps; then switch to the other foot.

Week 4: 20 Reps
Week 5: 25 Reps
Week 6: 25 Reps

3. Bent Knee Calf Raises

Sitting on a sturdy chair, with ankle weights, keep your body straight. Lift only your heels off the floor until your ankles are fully extended, putting pressure on the balls of your feet; hold, then slowly return heels to the floor.

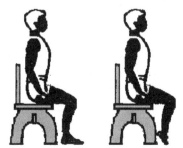

Week 7: 20 Reps
Week 8: 23 Reps
Week 9: 25 Reps

4. Elevated Calf Raises

Stand with your feet on an object such as a block, stool or stairs with your heels hanging just off the edge. Slowly lower the heels, as far down as comfortable. You should feel your calf muscles stretching. Then lift your ankles, placing your weight on the balls of your feet until your ankles are fully extended.

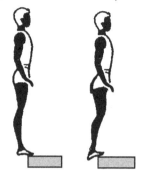

Week 10: 20 Reps
Week 11: 23 Reps
Week 12: 25 Reps

5. Rocking Calf Raises

Stand with your feet slightly apart. Lift your toes off the floor as high as comfortable, supporting your body weight on your heels. Then lift your heels off the floor until your ankles are fully extended to support your body weight on the balls of your feet.

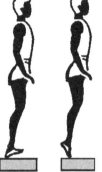

Week 13: 25 Reps
Week 14: 27 Reps
Week 15: 30 Reps

Group VI: Abdomen/ Hip Flexors

This group consists of exercises designed to strengthen the abdomen with special attention to the hip flexors. Strengthening the abdominal muscles is important in preventing back injuries.

1. Traditional Crunch

Lie on your back with your knees bent, feet on the floor, and your hands placed behind the neck.

Depending on your strength, the arms may be crossed over the chest or held over the head with elbows next to the ears (not thrown forward). Slowly roll up abdomen, bringing your shoulder blades off the ground; hold, and then slowly lower your shoulder blades to the ground. Inhale on your way up, exhale on your way down.

Week 1: 20 Reps
Week 2: 25 Reps
Week 3: 30 Reps

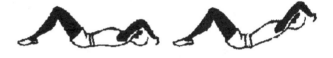

2. Raised Feet Crunches

Lie on your back with your knees bent, and hands behind the neck. Raise your feet off the floor until knees are perpendicular to the floor and hold them there throughout the exercise. Slowly crunch up, bringing your shoulder blades off the floor, hold, then lower your torso back to the ground. Inhale on your way up, exhale on your way down.

Week 4: 20 Reps
Week 5: 25 Reps
Week 6: 30 Reps

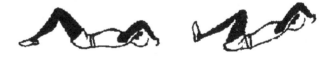

3. Sit ups

Lie on your back, with your knees bent, feet on the floor and your hands placed behind your neck. Keep elbows out to the side and not thrown forward. Raise your torso off the floor to bring your forehead to the knees. Fast up, slowly down. Inhale on your way up, exhale on your way down.

Week 7: 20 Reps
Week 8: 25 Reps
Week 9: 30 Reps

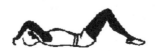 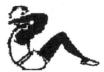

4. Convulsion

Lie on your back with your legs straight and arms straight on the floor above your head. In one movement, lift your arms, head and torso off the floor, along with your feet about one foot high above the floor. Flatten your lower back against the floor, hold for five seconds, then return to the starting position. Inhale on your way up, exhale on your way down.

Week 10: 20 Reps
Week 11: 25 Reps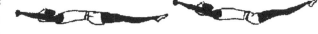
Week 12: 30 Reps

5. Front Scissor

Lie on your back, with your arms on the floor at your sides. Raise both feet about a foot off the floor, and move your legs in a scissor-like motion, keeping your feet off the floor. Make sure that your lower back is flattened against the floor throughout the movement.

Week 13: 20 Reps
Week 14: 25 Reps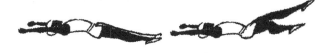
Week 15: 30 Reps

Group VII: Arms/ Biceps

This group consists of exercises primarily designed to strengthen the bicep muscles. The biceps need to be strong enough to counteract the strength of the triceps. They are opposing muscles. Strong biceps may protect the elbow from injuries related to hyperextension.

1. Biceps Curl

Stand with feet shoulders width apart, with dumbbells in hands, arms down at sides, and palms facing up. Bend your elbows and bring the dumbbells up to your shoulders, hold for 4 counts, then return to the starting position.

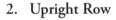

Week 1: 13 Reps
Week 2: 20 Reps
Week 3: 25 Reps

2. Upright Row

Stand with feet shoulder width apart, holding one dumbbell in each hand, in front of you, with thumbs facing each other. Bending your elbows, lift your upper arms straight out to the side, pulling the dumbbells straight up just until below chin level.

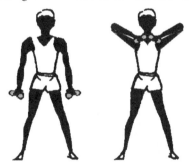

Week 4: 13 Reps
Week 5: 15 Reps
Week 6: 17 Reps

3. Hammer Curl

Stand with your feet shoulder width apart, holding one dumbbell in each hand, palms facing each other, elbows bent and at sides. Perform a curl, bringing thumbs to shoulders.

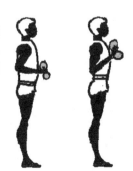

Week 7: 15 Reps
Week 8: 20 Reps
Week 9: 25 Reps

4. Biceps Curl

Repeat the exercise, with increased number of reps.

Week 10: 20 Reps
Week 11: 23 Reps
Week 12: 25 Reps

5. Upright Row

Repeat the exercise with increased number of reps.

Week 13: 20 Reps
Week 14: 23 Reps
Week 15: 25 Reps

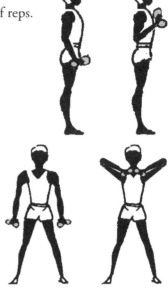

Group VIII: Back

This group consists of exercises designed to strengthen the back muscles.

1. Mule Kicks

With both hands and knees on the floor, and back rounded, pull one knee in toward chest, then push leg back while straightening knee and flattening back. When leg is extended, squeeze buttocks and lower abdominal muscles. Maintain a straight back during the movement, making sure not to rotate or twist your hips or lower back. Hips remain parallel to the floor. You can use ankle weights, depending on your strength. Perform the recommended number of reps; then repeat exercise with the other leg.

Week 1: 12 Reps
Week 2: 15 Reps
Week 3: 20 Reps

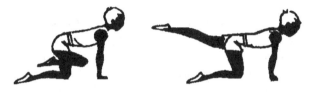

2. Convulsion

Lie flat on your stomach, arms out in front of you, close to your ears and palms facing down.

Legs are straight with feet together. To improve form and increase intensity, hold an ankle weight between your ankles. Lift your arms and legs off the ground, simultaneously and hold; then return to the starting position. Continue to look down during the movement to prevent overextending your neck. Squeeze your buttocks as you lift.

Week 4: 15 Reps
Week 5: 20 Reps
Week 6: 25 Reps

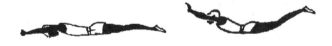

3. Shoulder Flexion Prone

Lie flat on your stomach, with arms overhead, close to your ears. Hold one dumbbell in each hand with your palms facing down. Rest your forehead on the floor (use a towel for support or comfort). Keep legs straight with feet together. Raise arms from floor and hold for five seconds; then return arms to the floor. Stabilize core by squeezing buttocks and contracting lower abdominal muscles.

Week 7: 10 Reps
Week 8: 12 Reps
Week 9: 15 Reps

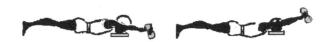

4. Back Extension

Lie flat on your stomach, with arms overhead, close to your ears. Legs are straight and slightly apart. Lift your chest off the floor as high as possible, while lifting your arms and head and hold; return to the starting position. Do not overextend your neck, and do not pull with your arms when lifting your chest off the floor. Keep core stabilized by squeezing buttocks and contracting lower abdominal muscles.

Week 10: 10 Reps
Week 11: 12 Reps
Week 12: 15 Reps

5. Cat Stretch

Place your hands and knees on the floor, with your back flat and parallel to the floor. Shoulders are squarely above your hands. Pull in your stomach while rounding your back, squeezing your abdominal muscles and your buttocks. Inhale and hold for one second. Then exhale and release the contraction until your back is fully arched. Tighten your back muscles. Hold for one second then repeat the entire exercise.

Week 13: 10 Reps
Week 14: 12 Reps
Week 15: 15 Reps

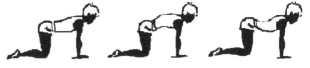

Group IX: Abdomen/Spine control

This group consists of exercises that are designed to help reduce back injuries. It is not just weak abdominal muscles that predispose the lower back to injury, but more specifically, weak lower abdominal muscles. The oblique abdominal musculature plays a vital role in protecting the lower back. Pelvic/spinal stabilization exercises are designed to give one the ability to use the muscles appropriately to protect the back and allow it to function normally. The pelvic tilt exercise is a basic example of this type of exercise.

1. Pelvic Tilts

Lie on your back with your knees bent, feet on the floor and your arms bent with your hands behind your neck. Flatten your back by tightening your stomach muscles and buttocks. Hold for five seconds, then relax and repeat.

Week 1: 10 Reps
Week 2: 12 Reps
Week 3: 15 Reps

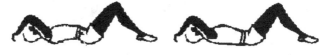

2. Cross - Knee Abdominal Crunches

Lie on your back on the floor, with your knees bent, feet on the floor and your hands behind your neck. Slowly raise your shoulders and upper back off the floor. Bring your right elbow towards your left knee, but do not touch. Hold at the top for at least one second; then slowly return to starting position. Repeat using left elbow and right knee.

Week 4: 30 Reps
Week 5: 35 Reps
Week 6: 40 Reps

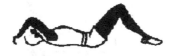

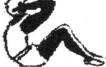

3. Bicycle

Lie on your back, and bend your hips and knees at a 90 degree angle so that your feet are in the air. Place your hands behind your ears, and slowly raise your shoulders and upper back off the floor. At the same time, lift your left leg to your chest and bring your right elbow to touch your left knee while you straighten your right leg keeping it a few inches off the floor. Lower your torso to the floor as you straighten your left leg and repeat the exercise this time drawing your right knee up as you crunch and bring the left elbow to touch the right knee; alternate from left to right, throughout the exercise.

Week 7: 30 Reps
Week 8: 35 Reps
Week 9: 40 Reps

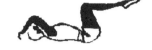 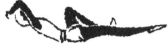

4. Inverted crunches

Holding a towel with your hands lie on your back with your legs straight and your arms on the floor above your had with palms facing up. Lift your arms, legs and hips off the floor, and bending at the wais and rounding your back, bring your legs in between your arms and with your feet over your head. Slowly return to the start up position.

Week 10: 12 Reps
Week 11: 15 Reps
Week 12: 20 Reps

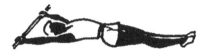 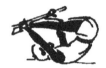

5. Hip Raises

Lie on back with your feet pointing up, and your arms resting at your sides, palms facing down. Raise feet up to the ceiling by contracting lower abdominal muscles and squeezing buttocks to rapidly curl the lower spine. Hips should rise up quickly off the floor. Hold the top position briefly and lower back down in a controlled two count.

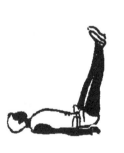 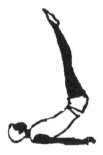

Week 13: 12 Reps
Week 14: 15 Reps
Week 15: 20 Reps

C. Cardiovascular Stamina

Cardiovascular exercise raises one's heart rate for a sustained period of time, and will increase stamina, burn calories, improve the function and efficiency of the heart, and lower blood pressure. Fast walking, jogging, biking, rope jumping, or just dancing to your favorite music are all examples of cardiovascular exercise.

D. Flexibility

Flexibility helps prevent injuries to the joints, by stretching the muscle fibers. The best time for really improving flexibility is when the muscles are warm and slightly fatigued, like after strength training. Flexibility exercises should follow strength training for several reasons:

- Muscles recuperate faster if they are stretched lightly. This is due in part to increased relaxation.
- Muscles have a tendency to become shorter during strength training. Stretching helps to negate this.
- Muscles are very warm and fatigued after strength training making them much easier to stretch.

1. Neck Roll

Stand up or sit down in a chair. Start by lowering your head down, with your chin as close to your chest, as comfortable. Slowly rotate your head towards your right shoulder with your ear close to the shoulder, then rotate back as far down as comfortable, feeling a full stretch in your neck; slowly continue to rotate your head to the left with your ear close to the shoulder, continue to rotate your head to come to the start up position. Repeat the exercise starting to rotate to the left.

2. Shoulder Roll

Stand with your hands at waist. Bring your shoulders up and roll them forwards in a circling motion, then reverse and roll your shoulders backwards. The goal is to get a full range of movement with your shoulders.

3. Shoulder Hyper Flexion

Stand with your legs slightly apart and your hands on the back of a sturdy chair. Bend forward at the waist, pushing your chest and head down as far as you can. Return to the start up position, and repeat the stretch for three to five times.

4. Shoulder Hyper Extension

Sit on the floor with your knees bent, feet on the floor and your arms straight, palms on the floor at the level of your hips, fingers pointing out. Walk your hands away from you, to reach as far out to the side as you can. Return to the starting position and repeat the stretch for three times.

5. Arms Scissor Stretch

Stand with your legs slightly apart and your arms straight in a lateral position with your palms facing down at shoulder level. Bring your arms forward and over your chest until they cross over as far as you can. Then open and bring your arms as far backwards as you can, pushing your chest out. Repeat ten times.

6. The Swimmer

Stand with your legs slightly apart and your arms down at your sides. Bring your arms forward, up, rotate backwards, down. Repeat ten times, then reverse and rotate your arms forward. On your back rotation open your chest wide, and on your front rotation slightly round your upper back.

7. Snake Stretch

Lie face down on the floor with your legs straight and together, with your hands by your chest, below your shoulders. Lift your chest and torso up into the air so that your upper body is nearly perpendicular to the floor. Keep your thighs on the floor, and your buttocks relaxed, as you lean backwards to stretch your abdominal muscles. Hold for two seconds then return to the starting position. Repeat five times.

8. Back and Hip Stretch

Sit on the floor with your legs stretched in front of you and toes pointing up. Place your right foot on the outside of your left knee, and your right hand behind your right hip. Bring your left arm straight up with fingers pointing to the ceiling and drop your chin down towards your chest. Take a deep breath. Then twist to the right and bring your left triceps to the outside of the right thigh, with your elbow pressing against your knee. Apply as much pressure as you can. Take a deep breath. Return to the starting position and repeat on the other side. Repeat the entire stretch three times.

9. Thigh Stretch

While standing, place your left hand on the wall for support. Bending your right knee, grab your right foot behind your back with your hand. Pull the foot towards your buttocks while lifting your chest forward and squeezing your shoulder blades together. Keep your knees together, and keep your abs pulled (contracted) the entire time. Hold for ten seconds. Repeat the stretch on the other side. Repeat the entire stretch twice.

10. Pike Stretch

Sit on the floor with your legs stretched in front of you, toes pointing up. Lift your arms overhead, and bend forward at the waist, with your hands reaching as close as possible to your ankles. Hold stretch for ten seconds then return to starting position. Repeat the exercise five times. Keep your legs straight throughout entire exercise.

11. Hips and Hamstring Stretch

Stand with your feet flat on the floor. Bend forward at your waist, while bending one knee. Let your upper body hang down, relaxed to release all the tension; alternate bending one knee while keeping the other leg straight. Stretch each side for ten seconds.

How to Exercise

If you never followed an organized exercise regimen, and/or you are not currently physically active, you must begin slowly; then gradually increase the intensity and duration of your workouts. For the first two weeks, you will start with walking to prepare your body for more intense activities. During the first week, begin by walking at your own pace for 30 minutes in the morning. Then in the second week, walk in the morning and evening for 30 minutes, at your own pace. At this point, you should be ready to introduce strength training. In the first six weeks of strength training, I recommend that you start with only two strength training sessions a week. After the six weeks, increase the frequency to three days a week.

If you are not new to exercise, and your fitness level and medical condition allows, then begin with three days of strength training per week. Follow the strength training circuit and flexibility exercises outlined below, performing the recommended number of reps for each week, beginning with week one. Below is a recommendation on how you should alternate your exercises throughout the week.

Day 1: Cardio

Walk in the morning for 30 minutes at your own pace.
If possible increase the peace almost to a fast walk.

Day 2: Strength Training

Warm-up:10 minutes of fast walking. Keep the peace of your walk to a çomfortable level.

Strength training circuit: 20 minutes; go through the circuit twice.

Flexibility/ stretch exercises: 5-10 minutes; follow the exercises listed in the flexibility section.

Day 3: Cardio

Walk in the morning for 30 minutes, at your own pace, increasing the pace to a fast walk, if possible (at a comfortable level).

Day 4: Strength training

Warm-up: 10 minutes of fast walking.

Strength training circuit: 20 minutes; go through the circuit twice.

Flexibility/stretch exercises: 5-10 minutes; follow the exercises listed in the flexibility section.

Day 5: Cardio

Walk in the morning **and** evening for 30 minutes per walk.

Day 6: Cardio

Choose one listed

Day 7: Cardio

Walk in the morning **and** evening for 30 minutes per walk

After six weeks or later, this is how your workout week should look:

Day 1: Cardio

Walk in the morning **and** evening for 45 minutes.

Day 2: Strength Training

Warm up: 10 minutes of fast walking. Keep your pace at a comfortable level at all times.

Strength training circuit: 20 minutes; go through the circuit 3 times.

Flexibility/ stretch: 5-10 minutes; follow the exercises listed in the flexibility section.

Day 3: Cardio

Walk in the morning **and** evening for 45 minutes.

Day 4: Strength training

Warm-up: 10 minutes of fast walking.

Strength training circuit: 20 minutes; go through the circuit 3 times.

Flexibility/stretch: 5-10 minutes; follow the exercises listed in the flexibility section.

Day 5: Cardio

Walk in the morning **and** evening for 45 minutes

Day 6: Strength Training

Warm-up: 10 minutes of fast walking.

Strength training circuit: 20minutes; go through the circuit 3 times.

Flexibility/stretch: 5-10 minutes; follow the exercises listed in the flexibility section.

Day 7: Cardio

20 -30 minutes, your choice of activity.

Remember that *you* will ultimately determine when you are ready to increase your work out. This will be based on whether you were new to exercise, as well as your current fitness and health. The six weeks time frame that I prescribed is simply a recommendation. It is more or less the average period of time needed to increase one's fitness level. If you feel comfortable doing the strength training exercises, and you have no difficulty performing them, you are ready to increase your work out. On the other hand, if after six weeks you are still having a difficult time performing the strength training exercises, give yourself more time until you feel ready. Just listen to your body, and you will know if and when you are ready. Also, make sure that on the days that you do strength training that you do not skip the warm-up. The warm-up will increase your heart rate and the temperature of your muscles, preparing them for exercises that follow, making them more viscous and less susceptible to injuries. If you do intense cardio exercise such as running, start slowly, then increase your pace, and follow with a cool down by slowly reducing your pace. Avoid stopping abruptly to reduce injury or muscle soreness.

Wherever You Are Exercises

The strength training exercises and stretches that follow can be done anywhere, whether you at work, sitting at your desk, or walking around. You can also do them at home while cleaning, doing laundry, cooking, watching TV, or reading a book. This approach is easy, convenient, and does not require a lot of time. Not only will you burn more calories throughout the day, but you will also shape up and improve your blood flow. *Your muscles will be the only ones working, just by contracting and relax them.* Correctly performing the strength training and flexibility exercises, will ensure that your muscles are exercised through the contractions and small movements. Not only will the muscles be worked during these exercises, but you will also become more aware of your muscles by isolating them, including those that you do not use everyday. This awareness, in turn, will allow you to maximize your workout by using the right muscles for each exercise, and reduce stress to muscles while you exercise.

1. Biceps Curl

Sitting on chair with your back pressed against the back of the chair, or while standing, bend your arms and press your elbows against your waist, with your hands close-fisted at the level of your elbows. Bring your fists at the level of your shoulder, contracting your biceps, hold; then return slowly to the starting position. Repeat five times.

2. Triceps Push- down

Stand with your legs slightly apart, arms straight at your sides, and your hands closed-fisted. Bring your arms straight in front of you with your fist at shoulder level. Bring your arms down and back just passing your hips, keeping your arms close to your body. Contract your triceps, hold, then relax and return to the starting position. Repeat five times.

3. Chest contraction

While sitting on a chair or standing, bend your arms and bring your hands in front of you at chest level. Shut your hands together, with only finger tips touching. Press your hands firmly against each other and contract your chest, hold, then relax. Repeat five times.

4. Good posture

Sitting, standing, or walking, maintain the alignment of your spine by periodically tightening your stomach muscles and buttocks. Hold for five seconds, relax, and repeat. Keep your neck and shoulders back relaxed and away from your ears to further elongate your spine.

5. Neck Roll

This exercise can be performed while standing or sitting. Begin by lowering your head down with your chin as close to your chest as comfortable. Slowly rotate your head towards your right shoulder with your ear close to the shoulder, then rotate back as far down as comfortable, filling a full stretch in your neck; slowly continue to rotate your head to the left with your ear close to the shoulder, continue to rotate your head to come to the start up position. Repeat the exercise starting to rotate to the left.

6. Shoulder Roll

Stand with your hands at waist. Bring your shoulders up and roll them forwards in a circling motion, then reverse and roll your shoulders backwards. The goal is to get a full range of movement with your shoulders.

7. Bent Knee Calf Raises

Sitting on a sturdy chair, keep your body straight. Lift only your heels off the floor until your ankles are fully extended, putting pressure on the balls of your feet, hold; then slowly return heels to the floor. Repeat five times.

8. Rocking Calf Raises

Stand or sit with your feet slightly apart. Then lift your heels off the floor until your ankles are fully extended to support your body weight on the balls of your feet. Then return the heels to the floor and lift your toes off the floor; repeat.

9. Outside Calf Rises

Sit on a chair with your back straight, and chin relaxed. Legs are bent at a 90 degree angle with feet on the floor. Turn your toes in and heels out, and lift your heels of the floor while tightening the small side calf muscles. Hold for 3 seconds; then return to the starting position. Repeat five times.

10. Leg extensions

Sit on a sturdy chair with your back straight against the back of a chair. Slowly lift both feet until your legs are fully extended, contracting your thigh muscles. Pause, then slowly lower your feet down to the initial position. Repeat ten times.

11. Nice Thighs

Sit on a chair with your back, straight legs bent at 90 degrees angle, with your feet on the floor. Slowly raise your right leg straight in front of you while tightening your thigh, then slowly bend your leg back while still maintaining your foot off the ground, then straighten again. Repeat 15 times. Repeat exercise on other leg.

12. Hip extender

Sit on a chair with your back straight, chin relaxed, legs bent at a 90 degree angle, with feet on the floor. Lift your left foot off the floor, extending it slightly off the chair. Move your leg from the front to the side as far as you can, then return to the front position. Focus on tightening your thigh muscles when moving your leg to the side, and your inner thigh muscle when returning to the front position. Keep your back straight and your stomach tight. Repeat the exercise on the other leg. Repeat the exercise five times, alternating legs.

13. Inner thighs

Sit in a chair with your back straight, chin lined up so that your spine is straight, legs bent 90 degrees with your feet on the floor. Bring your legs together and squeeze your inner thighs while pushing your knees one against each other. Hold for 5 seconds, relax and repeat for five times.

14. Quads

Sit on a chair with your back straight, chin relaxed, legs bent at a 90 degree angle, with feet on the floor. Cross your right leg over left knee, while pushing your right leg against your left knee. Tighten your quad muscle and hold for 3 seconds. Alternate legs and repeat the exercise five times.

15. Hamstring Curls

Stand with your hands on the back of a chair or a wall for support. Slowly bend one leg and bring up your heel as close as you can to your buttocks. Keep toes pointing down; hold; then return to the starting position. Repeat the exercise with the other leg. Repeat ten times on each leg.

16. Nice buttocks

While sitting, standing, or walking, squeeze your buttocks to tighten, hold, then relax and repeat as many times and/or as often you can.

17. Modified Crunches

Sit on a sturdy chair with your back placed firmly against the back of the chair. Place your hands on the chair by the sides of your legs. Keeping your arms straight and pressing down with your hands, slightly lift your heels off the floor, bringing your knees up, tightening your abdominal muscles and buttocks. Hold; then relax. Repeat ten times.

18. The Lifter

Sit on a chair with your back straight, chin relaxed, legs bent at a 90 degree angle, with feet on the floor. Arms should be straight by your side with hands on the side of the chair. Push down with your hands, while tightening your stomach muscles, to slightly lift your buttocks off the chair. Depending on your strength, you can lift your feet of the floor, or keep your toes on the floor. Slowly return back to the starting position, relax and repeat. Make sure that you tighten your arms and squeeze in your stomach. This exercise works your stomach muscles and triceps.

19. The Twister

Sit on a chair with your back straight, chin relaxed, legs bent at a 90 degree angle, with feet on the floor. Raise your arms out to the side and slowly twist your trunk to the right, maintaining a straight back and tightening your stomach. Return to the starting position, and twist again to the left side. Repeat the exercise five times on each side.

20. The Bender

Sit on a chair with your back straight, chin relaxed, legs bent at a 90 degree angle, with feet on the floor. With your arms straight and at your sides, slowly bend your trunk to the right while maintaining a straight back and tight stomach. Return to the starting position; then bend to the other side. Repeat five times on each side.

21. Breathing

Sit on a chair with your back straight, legs bent, and feet on the floor. Inhale, while tightening your abs, exhale, and relax your abs. Repeat ten times. This exercise will help you with your breathing techniques while exercising. Most people tend to hold their breath when tightening their muscles. This is incorrect. Breathing properly while exercising ensures that you maximize the amount of oxygen your heart receives during aerobic activity.

22. Back and Chest Stretch

Sit on a chair, or stand up, with your arms in front. Lift your arms up and back, opening your chest and arching your back. Hold for two seconds then return to the starting position. Repeat three times.

There are many strength training and flexibility exercises to choose from, many of which can be done wherever you are. For this book, I chose those that I found to be most beneficial, easy to perform, and that addresses all major group muscles. Whether you are a diabetic or not, or if you just need to lose weight, exercising will add lean muscle through strength training, work your heart through cardiovascular training, and add flexibility through stretching. In addition, exercising will help you burn fat, as well as calories throughout the day, reduce stress, and most importantly, improve your overall health and wellbeing. Therefore, be sure to incorporate exercise into your daily routine, walk as much as you can, and do strength training. There is no excuse to not exercise, because with my exercise, you can exercise wherever you are.

Chapter Eight

STARTING THE DIET

Armed with the knowledge of Type 2 Diabetes, our body, its functions and contribution of foods, I was ready to start my husband's diet. The first thing on the list was to go grocery shopping. I spent hours in different stores, looking for the first time at each and every product on the shelves, carefully reading the labels and writing down every product that contained less fat, fewer or no carbohydrates, high fiber, and those that contained little or no sugar.

> ❖ In appendix 4 I listed all the products that I used in my recipes.

I was very surprised when I realized the number of available products that I had ignored for so many years. The variety of products made me feel a little bit better, because I knew it would be hard to have my husband stick to the diet since he was a picky eater. He didn't like to eat the same foods all the time. I knew I had to be very creative with the food itself and with the presentation.

Though I like to cook, time was my biggest enemy, due to my busy schedule mornings and evenings working at the gym. I definitely didn't have much time to spare, but we were desperate and I was willing to do whatever it took to help him feel better. I went to Gordon Food Service, also called GFS, where I found plastic containers in all sizes, perfect for breakfast, lunch, snacks, and dessert. This helped me to be able to make and store food for two or three days at a time, as well as divide it into healthy portions. I labeled the food for each day, for breakfast, mid-morning snack, lunch, mid-afternoon snack, and dinner. I also made sure that there was no other food in the house that would tempt him. I knew that in order for him to eventually reduce his appetite, have fewer cravings, and lose weight, he would need to eat smaller portions throughout the day.

As mentioned before, our first objective was to detoxify or cleanse his body, and reset his biological clock. Despite all the negative things that I read about the detoxifying diets, I personally disagree. I don't believe that they are totally useless. If you have diabetes or you are dealing with obesity, your organs don't function the way they should. Detoxifying cleanses your organs and restarts them to function the right way. In addition, they will teach you to no longer crave carbs and sweets. As a result, the must-have sensation disappears. There is a large variety of detox-diets on the market such as liquid diets, pills or vitamins with the role of detoxifying different organs. However, I decided that it would be best for my husband Marian to have a food-based detox-diet. At the same time, I had to keep in mind that he was a diabetic and that I didn't know the side effects of any of the detox-diets available on the market.

I made the meals using the following three guidelines:

- Do not use or prepare foods that contained "bad," unhealthy fats.
- Meals were to contain low amounts of carbohydrates and lean proteins.
- Meals were to contain more fresh salads and raw vegetables.

I also used more of the ingredients that I found to be beneficial in helping with his condition. I knew that it wasn't going to be easy for him to adjust, since his prior diet was different. Nevertheless, he was in a desperate situation since nothing else was working, and was willing to do whatever it took.

I was not concerned about this new diet being too strict. I knew for a fact that it would be healthy, and it would include all of the nutrients required for our body to function properly. I also knew it would be safe for him to keep it for a month or so, since this detox phase was just the first step in achieving a healthy way of eating and living. Furthermore, he needed to lose at least 10 to 15 pounds, being that losing weight has a great influence on improving insulin sensitivity. Sometimes a very restrictive diet can deprive the body of some of the essential minerals and vitamins. These diets should be used for only a short period of time as jumpstart.

I remember that when I was a gymnast some of my team mates were on a restricted diet for few years, and they were in perfect health. In fact, a few years ago, while at dinner after an out of town competition with the girls' team, one of the team mothers was having just a plain dinner salad. I asked her why, since she looked fairly thin and lean to me. She told me that she used to be really fat three years ago, and since she had been on a restricted diet of mostly salads, lean meat and fruit, she lost 60 pounds and never felt better.

To succeed on any diet, the food must taste good, have enough variety, be fulfilling, and not give a sense of being deprived. Change your mindset when beginning your diet. Rather than thinking "diet," think "healthy eating" instead. Consider that you are trying to find a new way to treat yourself (by sampling new foods), as though you are dining a la carte. Seeing the results that you hope to achieve will fuel the motivation to keep you going! Believe me when I say that only the first few days are hard! In fact, after few weeks you will begin to feel as if this has always been your natural eating habit.

MEAL PLAN

The following is the meal plan that my husband followed at the beginning of his diet. I call it the detox-stage. You can make your own meal plan by combining the recipes any way that's convenient for you, without affecting the results. Choose any of the breakfasts, lunches, dinners, and snacks for any given day, and repeat the ones you liked the most while skipping the ones you don't. I made my recipes by trying different things, and by altering the ones I already knew.

For the purposes of this book, I kept only those recipes that testers liked and those that were effective in lowering my husbands' sugar level. In this initial phase, he didn't have any bread, grains, or fruits, and no flour was added to any of the recipes. All dairy products contained 2% fat (I found that their sugar content was lower than the fat-free ones). The only vegetables that were used were those with low-carbohydrates content, and no sugar or sweeteners were used in any of the recipes.

Monday

Breakfast: 2 Vegetable Quiche; sugar-free tea.

Snack: 1 stick, 2% reduced-fat mozzarella cheese.

Lunch: 2 tuna salad stuffed tomatoes served over bed

of romaine lettuce with 2 tablespoons lemon juice.

Snack: Fat-free Hummus with fresh celery.

Dinner: ½ Grilled chicken breast; 3 Zucchini Patties, Red Cabbage Salad.

Dessert: 1 cup Sugar-free gelatin

Tuesday

Breakfast: Baked omelet; sugar-free bilberry tea.

Snack: ½ cup 2% reduced-fat cottage cheese and grape tomatoes.

Lunch: Italian salad

Snack: 1-2 wedges light Laughing Cow cheese with red bell pepper slices

Dinner: Eggplant Moussaka; Roasted Peppers Salad.

Dessert: 1 cup sugar-free gelatin.

Wednesday

Breakfast: Turkey breast frittata; Sugar-free coffee.

Snack: Fat-free hummus with fresh celery.

Lunch: 2 Chicken salad stuffed tomatoes served over a bed of romaine lettuce with 2 teaspoons Vinaigrette Sauce.

Snack: 1 stick 2% reduced-fat mozzarella cheese

Dinner: Cod and Cabbage Delight.

Dessert: Sugar-free gelatin.

Thursday

Breakfast: 2 Egg white roll-ups; sugar-free bilberry tea.

Snack: ½ cup Cottage Cheese Delight; cherry tomatoes.

Lunch: Chef' salad, with 2 tbsp. vinaigrette sauce.

Snack: 3 slices fresh mozzarella cheese; red bell pepper slices.

Dinner: Broccoli soup; 2 Tuna rolls, Cabbage Salad.

Dessert: 1 cup sugar-free gelatin.

Friday

Breakfast: Vegetable omelet; sugar-free coffee.

Snack: 1-2 wedges Light Laughing Cow cheese; fresh celery.

Lunch: Chicken Salad with 2 tbsp. vinaigrette sauce.

Snack: ½ cup Part-skim ricotta cheese; sliced radishes.

Dinner: 2 Stuffed peppers; mixed greens
salad with vinaigrette sauce.

Dessert: 1 cup sugar-free gelatin dessert.

Saturday

Breakfast: Mushroom Omelet; sugar-free bilberry tea

Snack: 1 stick, 2% reduced-fat mozzarella cheese.

Lunch: ½ Grilled chicken breast; Spinach Salad.

Snack: ½ cup Fat-free hummus with fresh celery.

Dinner: Cod stew; Radicchio salad with 2 tbsp. Vinaigrette Sauce.

Dessert: 1 cup sugar-free gelatin dessert.

Sunday

Breakfast: 2 Turkey Burgers with mushroom salsa; sugar-free bilberry tea.

Snack: ½ cup 2% reduced-fat cottage cheese with grape tomatoes.

Lunch: Savory Shrimp; Spinach salad I.

Snack: ½ cup Part-skim ricotta cheese; green bell pepper slices.

Dinner: Salmon Delight; Eggplant and bell pepper casserole; Endive salad with vinaigrette sauce.

Dessert: 1 cup sugar-free gelatin dessert.

This meal plan should give you an idea of how to alternate servings of fish and meat through the day and week. Also, this meal plan contains at least two servings of raw vegetables per day. You can have unlimited quantities of those raw vegetables each day, as a snack or salad. Browse through the recipes and make your own meal plan, following the same rules:

- Low-fat
- Low-carbohydrates
- Alternate servings of meat and fish
- Include at least one salad a day
- Minimum of two servings of raw vegetables per day

Eating raw vegetables will give you the full benefit of its vitamins and minerals content. We all know too well by now that the cooking process destroys some of the vitamins and minerals in vegetables and fruits. Keep few things in mind:

- Eat every day at the same time
- Do not skip meals
- Eat only until you are satisfied not stuffed

The biggest mistake that one can make is to skip meals while on a diet. Skipping meals will not help you lose weight. On the contrary, your body senses a starvation stage and will preserve all the stored energy in the form of stored fat, lowering your metabolism. Also, when you do finally eat, you may tend to overeat. By eating smaller portions more often, you will make less insulin at a time, and reduce the cravings for more food in the hours to come. Also, when you eat small portions, and at the same time, your body knows that food is on the way, and your metabolic rate increases. In turn, you will burn the stored fat more efficiently.

Surprisingly, my husband followed the plan easily. The variety kept him from having to repeat the same meals too often, so he didn't get bored with the meals. He didn't feel hungry either. After the first two weeks his portions tended to reduce in size. In this initial phase, I didn't require him to monitor his sugar level in the morning because I knew he expected quick results, and would give up if he did not see a big difference.

After one month and 18 pounds lighter, he went back to the doctor to have his blood work done. The results were outstanding!

❖ See appendix 5 for the blood work results.

The doctor was amazed. He asked him what he done. When he found out that he was on a diet that I created for him, he told him to keep going because it was working! We were so happy! For the very first time in many years his glucose was 111 mg/dL and his triglycerides were down to 600 mg/dL.

Yes, he was still taking the highest dosage of medication Glugophage 1000 mg. 2 times a day and Glyburide 10 mg. 2 times a day, but for the first time his sugar level went down! His triglycerides were still high but no comparison to where it was previously, at 2000 mg/dL. It's working, and I felt like I was in heaven! He was happy, and more determined then ever to keep going.

—————— Chapter Nine ——————

LIGHTS AT THE END OF THE TUNNEL

Getting the sugar level under control

We had so much hope! As mentioned before, we started this endeavor with the intent of seeing if he could reduce, or eliminate his medication. We also wanted to see if he could control his sugar level or even improve his condition by using the foods to his advantage. Even though, I was skeptical at the beginning, now, I saw the light! I knew we had hard work ahead of us, but we had a reason to believe it could be achieved.

Finding the Right Diet

Now was the time to move one step forward, and find out how each food affected his body, metabolism, and glucose level. In order to do that, my husband had to take his sugar level before breakfast, morning snack, lunch, afternoon snack, and dinner. I think we were the best clients for the testing strips! Nevertheless, it was painful and inconvenient, but it was the only way to find out his body's response to different foods.

Monitoring his sugar level so closely, helped me eliminate the vegetables, fruits, and grains that had an effect on increasing his sugar level. I kept the ones that had little or no effect on increasing the sugar level. I also encourage you to monitor your sugar level in response to the foods you eat. This is the only way for you to know which fruits, vegetables, and grains are right for you to keep. It is also the only way to know which quantities (servings) are right for you. It all depends on how severe your situation is, and how much damage has already been done by diabetes.

With the knowledge that diabetics could not process carbohydrates and fats properly, I had to pay close attention to the foods that I included in his diet, and account for all carbohydrates, regardless of their form. For instance, 4 grams of carbohydrates will still be 4 grams, whether we get that from table sugar, or from carrots.

Every carbohydrate is processed and converted to glucose, and that's how it enters the blood stream. The critical questions now are:

- How fast are those carbohydrates broken down?
- How fast do they enter the blood stream?
- How this process affects the sugar (glucose) level?

With my husband having tried so many diets previously, I came across the concept that it was OK for diabetics to have sugar, as long as it is consumed in moderation. I now strongly disagree with that concept, because when my husband ate table sugar or in the form of honey, jelly, and cookies, his sugar level escaladed very quickly and for long periods of time. I also failed to understand *what "moderation" was, and what moderation was for each individual?* My own experiment left me with only one conclusion: the slower the absorption of the carbohydrates, the better it is for diabetics.

Why making your own menu?

I remember how excited and hopeful we were when we first ordered the precooked meals from one of the many diet providers on the market. The meals were specifically cooked and portioned for diabetics (according to the advertisement). Plus, it was convenient with no hassle in the kitchen or at the groceries stores. Depending on who the diet provider is, you can get your food for at least three days at the time. We got ours for one month at the time. Also, it is advertised to cost less money. Saving time, money, and getting the right food for diabetics, sounds like a win-win situation!

One of the things I decided was to try some of the meals before I gave them to my husband. Even though, I wasn't a diabetic I could use the convenience of precooked meals. In addition, both of us eating the same meals would make it easier for my husband to keep on the diet. But when I opened the cans or packages that contained our daily meals, I honestly didn't feel like trying them. The food was not appealing at all! And, though I pushed myself to try it (repeating in my mind that it was good for my health), after the first bite, I wanted to stop. The food didn't taste good! Maybe this was the message that if you don't like it you don't eat it, and the problem is solved. Besides the fact that the food wasn't appealing, and the portions were small, you also felt hungry shortly after eating. The carbohydrates and sugar content was also high for diabetics. What a disappointment that was.

Monotony, I believe is one of the reasons why most diets are unsuccessful. We get bored eating the same food every day for long periods of time. Also, lack of presentation and taste reminds us that we are on a diet. It could be quite depressing to think that you could be on a diet for the rest of your life, and have so many foods forbidden to you. I find that the more you know certain foods are restricted, the more you are going to want them!

I spent many hours in the kitchen. I had to create all kinds of recipes in order to have a large variety of meals. I also had to design a diet that would be healthy, provide all the nutrients, vitamins, and minerals that our body needs in order to function properly. Considering that my husband was a picky eater, I had to make foods that would taste good, be tempting, and easy to prepare. After all, this was going to be the diet that he would be on for the rest of his life.

I knew that changing the way the foods were prepared would give me the variety I was looking for. And it would make more foods accessible and in compliance with the guidelines for Type 2 diabetes:

- Low-fat
- Low-carbohydrates
- Low-starches
- Sugar-free or low-sugar
- High-fiber
- Rich in good fats(omega 3)

I didn't want my husband to think he was on a diet. I wanted him to consider this a better way to eat and a better way to live. What could be better then fresh cooked meals prepared right in front of your eyes, with appetizing fresh aroma that filled the kitchen? These foods had no preservatives, dehydration, and weren't processed, everything fresh. Gourmet food every day in your own kitchen! What more could you ask for?

Becoming the Chef

I was really enjoying this new journey. I felt like a real chef! My husband bought me all these fancy, yet useful, kitchen accessories. He bought a food processor, slicer, dicer–you name it, and we had it. My kitchen looked really professional. Thank God, we had a big kitchen with lots of counter space to fit everything. I was like a kid with lots of new toys, and ready to play!

The thought of creating new recipes was overwhelming at the beginning. Even though I had been cooking since childhood, and liked to cook, I wasn't a chef! I didn't know where to begin. But, I took a deep breath, and took one step at the time. I cannot say that it was easy or hard, it was time consuming. I initially began by changing the recipes I already knew, which led me onto creating knew ones. I changed the ingredients, the seasonings, and the way the food was prepared. I did a lot of mix and match, and tried some daring combinations. Some foods turned out to be good, and some went straight to the garbage. I only kept the recipes that he liked and incorporated them into his diet, and this book. I had my daughter and some of my friends try them also. I wanted to make sure the food I was creating was appealing and good, besides being just healthy.

The foods that I prepared for my husband's diet were grilled, boiled and steamed. Everything was low-fat, low-sugar or sugar-free, low-carbohydrate, and high in fiber. His daily menu was balanced, and comprised of unlimited quantities of vegetables (as much as he wanted to eat), and servings of meat, fish, dairy products, and fruits. I sparingly introduced small quantities of whole wheat pasta and rice into his diet. I even tried mashed potatoes and white rice, just to see how his body responded. He had three meals a day and two snacks, one in the morning and one in the afternoon. He also ate at the same time each day. I introduced some cereals for breakfast, flaxseed crackers and fruits for snacks and dessert. While the breakfasts and lunches were richer, the dinners which consisted mainly of different salads and sometimes desserts were light. I adjusted the menu, meals and quantities, throughout the day and week, based on his body response to the different foods. For instance, if after one particular meal his sugar level was high, the next meal was light, and with lots of vegetables.

> ❖ Appendix 6 contains a detailed daily menu that my
>   husband followed for the next twenty days, as well as
>   the sugar level response to the foods he ate.

You can follow the same daily menu, or you can create your own based on your own taste, and follow the same guidelines with plenty recipes to choose from in the Recipes chapter.

Eureka!

We were finally able to have the sugar level under control. We did it! I felt like jumping up and down like a kid. Is this good or what? My eyes could not believe that the numbers were within normal range. Even though at the beginning of his new diet they were a little bit higher then normal, ranging between 129 and 190, that was a lot better than the 300-400 range he had before. Sometimes the sugar level increased due to the foods he ate, but it came back to normal the next day, at times even before the next meal.

My husband was eating a wide variety of foods, and most importantly he did not feel like he was on a diet. He was no longer hungry between meals.

During the second phase of his diet, he lost another ten pounds. Though I was hesitant at first, his body responded positively to the new foods that I introduce in his diet. It included cereals, fresh fruits, sweet potatoes, and whole wheat flour in some recipes. I decided to keep white potatoes and white rice out of his diet since they caused such an increase in his sugar level. Perhaps if all goes well, he can limit mashed potatoes to holidays, or special occasions.

The results of this phase led me to believe that his body was starting to process foods and especially carbohydrates more efficiently. After all, maybe we did increase the insulin sensitivity. My husband was eating healthier then before, and he had lost a total of 28 pounds so far! He was exercising every day for 30 minutes before and sometimes after diner, depending on what time he got back from work. Above all, he was *feeling* better! He had more energy, and wasn't depressed. His overall quality of life improved as well.

I knew that we were definitely on the right track. Having the sugar level under control and pretty much stabilized, made me decide that it was time to take it one step further, and reduce the medication by half of the regular dosage.

──── Chapter Ten ────

VICTORY!

Journey to Being Medicine Free

It's Not Always Easy

I must admit, I was a little bit anxious. I know that we had the sugar level under control, but he was still taking a full dosage of medication. Nevertheless, we were ready for the next big step which was to observe the effects of reducing his medication to half the dose. After all, this was our big goal from the beginning—to reduce or even eliminate his medication.

When my husband started to feel better, some of his old cravings returned. He started to question why he couldn't have baked goods or bread, or even steak and potatoes every once in a while. His excuse was that he was getting bored. He argued that since we had the sugar level under control, certain foods shouldn't be a problem. I realized then, that he considered this diet a temporary solution, and that one day it would allow him to eat without restrictions.

We've all experienced frustration when something happens to us, and we all asked the eternal question, "*Why me?*" I knew he needed my support. I had to be strong and not let him give in. I told him to change the way he thought about food. I also told him to accept who he was, and just deal with it the same way he would with any other event in his life.

Getting his body to process foods better would take time. You cannot expect to eliminate a problem like Type 2 diabetes overnight, or even a year. It is a slow and progressive condition, resulting from years of poor metabolism and inadequate diets. There are no quick fixes and he of all people, should know this. I promised him that if everything went right, and his body began to process foods better, he would be able to have some of his old favorites again. We would introduce some breads and deserts into his diet, and make Sunday an "indulging" day.

Medication Reduced to Half Dose

I didn't change the diet again, only the medication. I made one change at the time. My husband took only half the dosage of his medication for the next twelve days. He had the same meals and snacks as before, around the same times. We continued to monitor his sugar levels as closely as before.

Everything was going great. Even on half of the medication, the sugar level was within normal range. I was right on target! Reducing the fat, substituting bad fats with good fats, eliminating processed carbohydrates, and increasing the vegetables (including the raw vegetables) in his diet, proved to be the keys to reducing his sugar level and keeping it under control. I now had real data to prove it.

> ❖ In appendix 6 you will find a detailed meal plan that my husband followed for twelve days, while on half dosage of medication, as well as the sugar levels.

After the first six days into this new phase of his diet, everything was going good. I kept the promise I made to my husband, and made Sunday the indulging day. After all, a promise is a promise. I did this for two reasons. First, to ease his frustration a little bit, and secondly, to see how his body would now react to different foods. I wanted to see in terms of how they affected his sugar level. Even though the meals on Sunday were scrumptious, I made sure the portions were smaller. He had his steak that he wanted for so long, shrimp chowder, bread and even ice cream. The sugar level did increase quite a bit, but it went back to a normal range the next day. That was a lot better than I expected, and it made me decide to keep the Sundays as the "indulging" days. You can choose your own indulging day, but make sure that it is only one day of the week, and the portions are small.

The next day he was back to his regular diet. Since everything was going in the right direction, we began to take his sugar levels only before breakfast, lunch, and dinner. We pretty much got all the answers that we needed.

Who Is He?

My husband was doing great and most importantly, he was feeling better. He lost his belly fat, and looked the same way he did when we first met. He was constantly getting compliments, and was looking younger as well! We all know that when we begin to get results and they are acknowledged by others, it's not only flattering, but it motivates us to keep going. He was no different. He was happy, his mood changed, his energy level went up, and he no longer felt urges for his old favorite foods. Not only did he change on the outside, but the changes within were even more profound. He changed the way he thought about food, diets, diabetes, and life in general. Food was no longer the center of his life, and was no longer his source of comfort. Instead, he cared about his body again, and was willing to do what was necessary to keep it going.

He developed new and healthy habits, and now had a new lifestyle. He also no longer dreaded having to exercise, but rather looked forward to it. One evening, we had to stay later then usual at the gym, so we got home really late and went straight to bed. The next morning he was not himself. When I asked him what was wrong, his reply stunned me, he said he didn't exercise last night, and he felt tired and sluggish. I couldn't believe this was my husband, the same one who had such a hard time in the beginning, even walking on the treadmill for twenty minutes.

This was the best time ever! It was also the time to pay the doctor a visit and have a lab test done to check on his cholesterol, blood pressure, and triglyceride levels. We got the results a few days later, and everything was within normal ranges. The doctor was amazed and pleased with Marian's results and encouraged him to keep going. Great! We agreed to do just that.

Medication Reduced to ¼ Dosage

It was time to take it one step further, and reduce the medication to a quarter of the dosage. I had my hopes up, and was confident, but still kept my fingers crossed. Would it really be possible to get him off medication? This question was stuck in my head. I knew that we had great results so far, but I still had some doubts. We all know what it feels like deep down inside, when we get so close to realizing our dream.

For the next two weeks he followed the same diet and exercise regimen, and he took only a quarter of his medication. I shouldn't even call it a diet anymore, since it was now our new way of eating. Like I said, it was like having gourmet food in your own kitchen. We continued to monitor his sugar levels as closely as before. I must admit, the first day I was nervous. But after I saw that the sugar level was within the normal range, I relaxed. I even introduce some new fruits into his menu, like fresh pear and fresh cantaloupe.

❖ A detailed daily menu and sugar level counts are listed in the Appendix 6.

The results were outstanding and we couldn't be any happier. We started with a full dosage of medication, and now we were on just a quarter of it, and his sugar level was within normal range. Medication no longer played an important role in controlling his blood sugar level! I had got the answer that I was hoping for. This was the reason I had started all my research and took us through our endeavor. I had the proof that you can control your diabetes with your diet.

Chapter Eleven

LIFE WITHOUT DIABETES

The Last Chapter of Our Journey

How Did We Get Here

I don't know how to emphasize more, the importance of knowing and understanding Type 2 diabetes. Knowing your foods, your body and its functions, empowers you to make the right decisions in regard to your diet. They are the tools you need to find out what works for you. Nobody can know your body better then you, if you're willing to take the time to listen to it! Also, you won't have to follow somebody else's diet, since there are no quick fixes, and one diet doesn't fit all. Monitoring your sugar level closely in response to the foods you eat, will help you design your own diet and ultimately control this condition. We did just that.

We were able to reduce my husband's medication because his body started to process foods more efficiently. And, that happened as a result of increasing insulin sensitivity through loosing weight, eliminating processed carbohydrates, and increasing the fiber intake. It was also achieved by eliminating the bad fats and by replacing them with good ones, and by increasing the vegetable intake in his diet.

We shared our results with his doctor, and after the Lab test results were in, he encouraged us to keep going.

It Will Be OK!

Here we were, facing the eternal question "To be or not to be?" We had our hopes up and we were ready for the best to come! I knew going into this that I had a back-up plan. Mainly, I knew he wasn't at risk. In the event of taking no medication his sugar level increased, we could always go back to a quarter of the dosage, which was working fine. I also told him, that no matter what, we should not allow ourselves to become disappointed. The worst that could happen was that he would have to stay on a quarter dose of his medication, perhaps for the rest of his life, or at least a little bit longer.

I urged him to look on the bright side since we've already accomplished so much! His sugar level, blood pressure, cholesterol, and triglycerides were all within normal ranges. He was a hundred times healthier than before. That was a huge achievement. He had lost weight, and was exercising on a regular basis. He looked and felt good, and best of all he changed his thinking about food. Food was no longer the central point of his life; sifted its meaning from comfort to that of an ally in controlling his diabetes. He was a new person with a new lifestyle! He was changed inside and out, and so was I.

The Last Big Step

Finally, we were one small step away from our biggest goal—completely eliminating medication from Marian's life. I felt the same way I used to feel when I was a gymnast at the last practice before a major competition. I knew I could do it because I was training and working hard. I had the skills, but there was always a "but" in the back of my mind. Just as I did then, I did now. I took a deep breath, and hoped for the best.

I knew that eliminating medication altogether would not mean "freedom" from diabetes in the real sense of the word, especially, in comparison to somebody who never had it, or was prone to having it. Type2 diabetes is a metabolic condition, and as long as you control it, and improve the way your body metabolizes food—from my point of view—that puts you in control. This also sets you free from medication and all the complications that this multifaceted condition generates.

This last step would be the biggest step we ever faced. I figured that if his sugar level went up on some days, we could always change the foods and observe the results as a first resort, and if needed, go back to medication second. He kept the same diet and exercise regime as before. He had his meals and snacks the same times, and monitored his sugar level as closely as before. Even though he was without medication, his sugar levels were still within normal ranges.

❖ In Appendix 6, you will find a detailed daily menu and sugar level counts.

We were determined, and we succeeded! My husband's body no longer needed medication to metabolize the foods he was eating. Can you imagine how we felt? This was a man who had struggled with diabetes for so many years, and had tried every diet that was on the market, and failed. Now he was in control. Not only was he in control of his diabetes, but also the way he perceived his priorities, his body, and the foods he ate. Though he's always had my support, he played the biggest role. He had the desire, strength, and determination that came from within.

You Can Do It

There is no better proof than our success in the importance of knowing your body, and how it responds to specific foods. Also, there is no better proof that one food pyramid and one diet does not work for everyone. When it comes to metabolism, one size definitely doesn't fit all. Despite my husband's success, we know that there will always be foods that he can't have without compromising his sugar levels. This is because his body simply can't metabolize them properly. However, not having them is a small price to pay for being in control of your condition.

To this day, this is the diet that my husband maintains. It took me two and a half years, from the day I began my research until I finished writing this book. During this time we maintained Sundays as our "indulging day," in which I made his favorite meal or desert. We also continue to enjoy our traditional foods on each holiday. Sometimes his sugar level would go up after such occasions, but he would immediately go back to his regular way of eating the next day, and no damage was done. He no longer ate big portions as before we started our endeavor. He felt satisfied with smaller portions and learned to stop eating after he felt full. His exercise regimen, which he continues up to this day, keeps him in shape and helps him burn more calories. It also increased his insulin sensitivity, thereby keeping his sugar level under control.

Whether you are a diabetic, struggle with high blood pressure or cholesterol, or just need to lose weight, there is only one answer, know your body and its functions. Also know your foods and the way they affect your body, and then design your own meal plan. Choose the foods and exercise regimen that fits your body and your lifestyle.

This book can assist you in your quest for better health by providing you with a real life depiction of how this can be accomplished. It provides plenty of exercises that you can choose from, according to your age, body and level of fitness. It also incorporates many recipes that are tasty, easy to prepare, and most of all, healthy. These are precisely the tools that you need to make it happen for you. **If we can do it, so can you!**

─── Chapter Twelve ───

RECIPES

BREAKFASTS

Mushroom Omelet

1 cup egg substitute
2 tablespoons fat-free milk
1 tablespoon Smart Balance spread
1 cup fresh mushrooms, sliced
Dash salt
Dash black pepper

Heat a skillet over low heat. Add the smart Balance spread and the mushrooms and cook until mushrooms are tender, for about ten minutes. Mix egg substitute, milk, salt, and pepper, and pour over mushrooms. Cover and cook on low heat until omelet is set.

Serves: 1

Sweet Potatoes Omelet

1 small sweet potato, shredded
1½ cup egg substitute
2 tablespoons fat-free milk
Dash salt substitute
Dash black pepper
½ teaspoon fresh dill, chopped

Spray a skillet with cooking spray, and place over low heat. Mix all the ingredients and add to the skillet. Cook uncovered till golden, flipping once.

Serve 2

Blueberry Bran Muffins

1 cup Fiber One bran cereal
1 cup ground flexed seed
1 ½ cup fat-free yogurt
1 cup egg substitute
½ cup egg whites
1½ teaspoon baking powder
1 teaspoon ground cinnamon
1 cup fresh blueberries
4 tablespoons Splenda sugar substitute

Preheat oven at 375 degrees. Beat the egg whites until stiff. Add sugar substitute 1 tablespoon at the time continuing to beat. Add the egg substitute, continuing to beat. Add yogurt, baking powder, cinnamon, and mix together until well combined. Fold in the bran cereal and ground flexed seed until well combined. Fold in the blueberries. Spray a 6-cup muffin pan with nonstick cooking spray. Divide mixture evenly between the muffin cups and bake for about 40 minutes or until a toothpick inserted in a middle of muffin comes out clean.

Serves: 6

Breakfast Parfait

1 cup fresh strawberries, sliced
1 cup low-fat, sugar-free yogurt
1 cup Fiber One bran cereal
½ teaspoon ground cinnamon
2 teaspoons sliced almonds

In a small bowl, put ½ cup strawberries, ½ cup yogurt, ½ cup bran cereal, the other ½ cup yogurt, ½ cup bran cereal, and ½ cup strawberries. Sprinkle cinnamon and almonds on top. Serve at once.

Serves: 1

Red Bell Pepper Omelet

1 cup red bell pepper, chopped
½ cup green onion, chopped
1 cup egg substitute
¼ cup 2% fat milk
½ cup 2 % fat mozzarella cheese, shredded
1 cup 98% fat-free ham

Spray a skillet with nonstick coking spray and place over medium heat. Add the green onion and red bell pepper to the skillet. Sauté for 5 minutes or until onion and pepper are tender. Set aside. Mix egg substitute and milk and add to the skillet. Cook until beginning to set, lift to allow uncooked eggs to run under. Add red bell pepper, green onion, mozzarella cheese, and ham. Cover and cook for 1 to 2 minutes or until cheese is melted. Serve folded over and garnish with 2% fat mozzarella cheese.

Serves: 2

Artichoke Quiche

1 can (14 ounces) artichoke harts rinsed and drained
2 tablespoons green onion with tops, chopped
1 garlic clove, minced
½ cup low-fat part-skim mozzarella cheese, shredded
½ cup 2% fat Monterey Jack cheese, shredded
1 tablespoon whole wheat flour
2 tablespoons ground flexed seeds
1½ cup egg whites
1 tablespoon cilantro, chopped
Dash black pepper
¼ teaspoon backing powder

Combine all the ingredients until well blend. Pour mixture into 6-cup baking pan coated with nonstick cooking spray, leaving ¼ of an inch from the top. Bake at 375 degrees for 30 minutes.

Serves: 6

Vegetable Quiche

¼ cup green onion, chopped
¼ cup red bell pepper, chopped
¼ cup celery, finely chopped
1 cup low-fat part-skim mozzarella cheese
1½ cup egg substitute
¼ teaspoon baking powder
Dash black pepper

Coat a skillet with cooking spray; sauté the onion, pepper, and celery until tender, over low heat. Mix the egg substitute, baking powder, black pepper, and cheese. Add the sautéed vegetables and mix well. Pour mixture into 6-cup baking pan coated with cooking spray and bake at 375 degrees for 30 minutes or until done.

Serves: 3

Bran Muffins

1 cup All Bran cereal
1 cup ground flexed seeds
½ teaspoon baking powder
2 cups egg substitute
½ teaspoon pure vanilla extract
1 teaspoon ground cinnamon

Mix well all the ingredients. Pour mixture into a 6-cup baking pan coated with cooking spray.
Bake in oven at 375 degrees for 30 minutes.

Serves: 6

Blueberry Muffins

1 cup ground flexed seeds
½ cup bran flour
1 tablespoon whole wheat flour
½ teaspoon baking powder
½ cup egg whites, beaten until firm
1 cup blueberries
¼ teaspoon rum extract
1½ cup egg substitute
2 tablespoons fat-free milk

Incorporate slowly egg substitute into firmly beaten egg whites. Mix milk, baking powder and rum extract. Mix together whole wheat flour, bran flour and flexed seeds. Incorporate the milk mixture and egg mixture into the flour, until well combined. Fold in the blueberries. Pour into 6-cup baking pan sprayed with cooking spray, leaving ¼ of an inch from the top. Bake at 375 degrees for 30 minutes.

Serves: 6

Cottage Cheese Pancakes

1 cup egg substitute
1 cup low-fat cottage cheese
1 cup low-fat sour cream
1 cup whole wheat flour
Sugar free syrup
½ teaspoon ground cinnamon

Blend all ingredients and fry as you would any pancakes. Serve with sugar free syrup.

Serves: 2

Baked Omelet

1½ cup egg substitute
½ cup fat-free milk
¼ cup green onion, chopped
¼ cup red bell pepper, chopped
¼ cup 98% fat-free turkey breast, chopped
¼ cup part-skim mozzarella cheese, shredded
Dash salt
Dash black pepper

Preheat the oven at 375 degrees. Mix all the ingredients until well blended. Spray a baking pan with nonstick cooking spray; pour mixture in the pan and bake for 25 minutes or until set.

Serves: 2

Apple Bran Muffins

1 cup medium green apple, shredded
½ cup ground flexed seeds
1 cup bran flour
1 tablespoon olive oil
¼ cup egg whites, stiffly beaten
¼ cup chopped walnuts
¼ teaspoon baking powder

Combine all the ingredients. Let it stand for 5 minutes. Mix together firmly. Spoon the mixture into 6-cup muffin baking pan, sprayed with cooking spray. Bake at 375 degrees for 25 minutes.

Serves: 6

Smoked Salmon Quiche

8 ounces smoked salmon, skinless and flaked
1 cup fat-free half-and-half
1 cup part-skim mozzarella cheese, shredded
1 cup egg substitute
½ cup green onion, chopped
1 tablespoon cilantro, chopped
Dash black pepper
¼ teaspoon baking powder
1 cup bran flour

Beat the eggs, half-and-half, and baking powder together. Add the salmon, onion, cheese, cilantro and black pepper. Mix well. Incorporate flour into mixture. Pour into 6-cups muffin pan sprayed with nonstick cooking spray. Bake at 375 degrees for 35 minutes, or until a knife placed in center of muffin comes out clean.

Serves: 6

Turkey Breast Frittata

3 slices 98% fat-free turkey breast, coarsely chopped
½ cup green onion, chopped
¼ cup celery, finely chopped
1½ cup egg substitute
¼ cup part-skim mozzarella cheese, shredded
Dash black pepper
Dash salt substitute

Spray a skillet with nonstick cooking spray and heat over medium heat. Add the onion, celery, and turkey, and cook covered until tender. Mix the egg substitute, milk, salt, and pepper. Add the egg mixture to the skillet, and cook covered, without stirring for about 7 minutes, or until eggs are almost set. Run a large spoon around the skillet edge, lifting eggs for even cooking. Sprinkle with cheese. Remove from heat, cover and let stand for 3 minutes until cheese melts.

Serves: 2

Egg Whites Roll Ups

1 cup egg whites
1 cup Canadian bacon, finely chopped
1 cup 2% fat Monterey Jack cheese, shredded
1 cup red bell pepper, finely chopped
¼ teaspoon salt substitute
Dash black pepper
1 tablespoon cilantro, finely chopped

Spray a skillet with nonstick cooking spray and place over medium heat. Mix the egg whites, salt, pepper, and cilantro. Pour a thin layer in the heated skillet and cook for 3 minutes; flip over and cook for additional 3 minutes. Transfer the thin egg whites layer to a plate. Repeat one more time. Sprinkle over each egg white layer ½ the bacon, ½ the red bell pepper, ½ the cheese. Fold into a roll (not to tight, not to loose).
Serve immediately.

Serves: 2

Vegetable Omelet

¼ cup green onion, chopped
¼ cup red bell pepper, chopped
¼ cup fresh mushrooms, chopped
¼ cup cherry tomatoes, chopped
1 garlic clove, minced
1 cup egg substitute
¼ cup fat-free milk
Dash salt
Dash black pepper
¼ cup 2% fat mozzarella cheese, shredded
1 tablespoon fresh dill, finely chopped

Spray a skillet with nonstick cooking spray. Add onion, garlic, red pepper, and mushrooms, cover and cook until tender. Add the tomatoes, uncover and cook stirring frequently, until all moister is gone. Meanwhile, mix the egg substitute, milk, salt, black pepper, and dill. Add the egg mixture to the skillet all at once. Cover and cook until almost set. Uncover and sprinkle the cheese on ½ of omelet, fold the other half over and cook for additional 2 minutes.

Serves: 2

Chicken Frittata

1 cup grilled chicken breast, chopped
1 cup sweet potatoes, shredded
2 cups stir-fry vegetables San Francisco style
1 cup egg whites
½ cup egg substitute
¼ cup 2% fat milk
1 teaspoon Dijon mustard
¼ teaspoon black pepper
1 garlic clove, minced
1 tablespoon cilantro, chopped
½ teaspoon salt substitute
½ cup part-skim mozzarella cheese, shredded

Preheat oven at 400 degrees. Spray a baking sheet with nonstick cooking spray. Spread potatoes on the baking sheet, sprinkle with salt and bake for 20 minutes or until potatoes are tender. Remove from the oven. Cook vegetables in a large skillet according to package directions. Mix egg whites, egg substitute, garlic, pepper, mustard, cilantro, and milk. Add potatoes and chicken breast to skillet and stir lightly. Pour the egg mixture over, in the pan. Cook covered over medium heat for 5 minutes or until the egg mixture is set. Uncover and sprinkle cheese on top. Place the skillet in the oven and bake for 5 minutes or until cheese is melted.

Serves: 2

Baked Green Beans Omelet

1pound green beans
1½ cup egg substitute
2 tablespoons 2% fat milk
1 teaspoon salt substitute

Boil the green beans for 10 minutes; drain and cut in 1 inch pieces. Mix egg substitute, milk and salt. Spray a baking pan with nonstick cooking spray. Place green beans into the pan, and pour the egg mixture over the beans. Bake in oven at 325 degrees until done.

Serves: 2

LUNCHES

Tortilla Roll Ups

1 (8 ounces) package fat-free cream cheese
8 ounces fat-free turkey breast lunch meat
1 green bell pepper, shredded
4 whole wheat tortillas

Spread a thin layer of cream cheese over each tortilla. Add 1 slice of turkey breast and 1 tablespoon of shredded green peppers. Roll tortilla tightly. Place seam side down on a plate. Chill at least two hours. Slice each roll into 1 inch slices forming a pinwheel. Arrange on a plate over lettuce and serve.

Serves: 4

Chicken Burritos

1 grilled chicken breast, thinly sliced
1 can (15 ounces) black-eyed peas, rinsed and drained
1 tablespoon mild green chilies, diced
3 garlic cloves, minced
¼ cup celery, finely chopped
1 cup cherry tomatoes, chopped
2 tablespoon fresh cilantro, chopped
6 whole wheat tortillas

Spray a skillet with nonstick cooking spray. Heat over medium heat; add garlic, celery and chicken breast to the skillet. Cook and stir continuously for 5 minutes. Stir in the beans, chilies, cilantro, and cherry tomatoes. Cook for additional 5 minutes. Spoon the chicken mixture evenly down center of each tortilla. Sprinkle the cheese evenly over the chicken mixture on each tortilla. Fold bottom end of tortilla over filling and roll up.

Serves: 6

Pickled Mushroom Salad

2 cans (6 ounces) mushrooms crowns, rinsed and drained
2 tablespoons red wine vinegar
1 tablespoon olive oil
1 small white onion, thinly sliced and separated in rings
Dash salt substitute
2 teaspoons fresh parsley finely chopped
1 teaspoon Dijon mustard
1 garlic clove, minced
8 romaine lettuce leaves

Mix vinegar, oil, garlic, salt, and parsley together in a saucepan, and bring to a boil. Remove from heat; add the mushrooms and toss to coat. Chill in a covered bowl for two hours before serving.
Drain and serve over the romaine lettuce.

Serves: 2

Creole Green Beans

1 pound fresh green beans
3 garlic cloves, minced
1 tablespoon white wine vinegar
1 tablespoon olive oil
1 tablespoon fresh dill, finely chopped
Dash salt substitute
Dash fresh ground black pepper

Cut the tips off the green beans, rinse and steam for 20 minutes. Spray a skillet with nonstick cooking spray; add the garlic to the skillet, place over low heat and cook for 5 minutes. Add the olive oil and the green beans and cook for additional 5 minutes. Remove from heat, add vinegar and dill, toss and chill for 1 hour before serving.

Serving suggestions: could be served by itself as a lunch, or as a side dish with grilled chicken breast as a dinner.

Serves: 2

Codfish Balls

½ pound frozen codfish fillet thawed
3 cups diced zucchini
¼ cup egg substitute
1 garlic glove minced
Dash salt substitute or to taste
Dash black pepper or to taste

Finely chop the codfish and mix with zucchini. Beat with the electric mixer and add egg substitute, salt and pepper. Beat thoroughly. Separate the mixture into golf size balls (about 1 tablespoon). Spray a pan with nonstick cooking spray, place over medium heat and heat thoroughly. Slightly flatten each ball and place it in the pan. Cook on each side until golden brown (about 6 minutes).

Serving suggestions: with zucchini patties, with sauce piquant over romaine lettuce, or garlic sauce.

Serves: 1

Tuna Burgers

1 pound fresh tuna
1 teaspoon soy sauce
½ teaspoon sesame oil
1 medium red onion
3 garlic cloves
1 teaspoon fresh ginger
¼ teaspoon red pepper flakes
Salt and ground black pepper to taste

Put all ingredients in a food processor, and process until well blend. Shape tuna mixture into equal size patties. Broil the patties for 3 to 5 minutes on each side or until patties are golden brown. Serve over a bed of romaine lettuce, top with refreshing salsa (see recipe).

Serves: 2

Greek Style Eggplant

1 medium eggplant
¼ cup egg substitute
1 medium white onion, finely chopped
1 garlic clove, minced
3 plum tomatoes, chopped
¼ cup pitted black olives, cut into small slices
Fresh parsley chopped
Pinch salt substitute
Dash black pepper

Cut the eggplant crosswise into ¼ inch rounds. Dip each eggplant round into egg substitute and place the rounds onto a nonstick cooking pan. Bake in the oven, until golden brown, flipping once. Meanwhile, sauté the onion and garlic, into a nonstick skillet, for 5 minutes, or until the onion is golden. Add tomatoes, salt, and pepper and cook for about 15 minutes on low heat, stirring occasionally. Put a generous tablespoon of sauce over each eggplant round, and top with black olives. Stack if necessary. Bake uncovered for ten minutes. Sprinkle with fresh parsley before serving.

Serves: 2

Cheese Eggplant

1 medium eggplant
1 cup 2% fat mozzarella cheese, shredded
Dash salt
Dash black pepper
Dash garlic powder

Cut the eggplant length wise into ¼ inch slices. Sprinkle each eggplant slice with salt, pepper and garlic, and grill on a sprayed with nonstick cooking spray, cooking sheet on high until golden brown, flipping once. Add a generous amount of cheese on each eggplant slice and grill for an additional 3 minutes or until cheese melts. Serve hot or cold.

Serves: 2

Cucumber Soup

1 medium cucumber
½ quart fat-free butter milk
2 tablespoons green onion, chopped
1 teaspoon salt substitute
¼ cup fresh parsley, chopped
Dash black pepper

Peel cucumber, remove seeds and grate. Put the cucumber in a soup bowl, add the remaining ingredients, and mix well. Cover and chill about 1 hour before serving.

Serves: 1

Gazpacho

2 cups low-sugar tomato juice
½ cup green bell pepper, chopped
½ cup cucumber, skinless, seedless, and chopped
1 garlic clove, minced
½ cup celery, chopped
8 cherry tomatoes, chopped
1 tablespoon white wine vinegar
1 tablespoon lemon juice
Dash salt substitute
Dash black pepper
1 tablespoon fresh parsley, finely chopped

Mix all the ingredients in a bowl and chill for about one hour before serving.

Serves: 1

Broccoli Soup

1(10 ounces) package frozen chopped broccoli
1½ cups fat-free milk
1 cup fat-free yogurt
2 tablespoon green onion, chopped
1 tablespoon chives, chopped
½ teaspoon salt substitute
Dash black pepper

Thaw the broccoli and place in the blender with 1 cup fat-free yogurt. Blend until well combined. Add the remaining ingredients, and blend until smooth, about 45-60 seconds. Chill for 1 hour before serving. Serve topped with parsley (optional).

Serves: 2

Tomato Soup

2 cups tomato juice
½ cup green onion, chopped
½ teaspoon ground nutmeg
2 tablespoons fat-free sour cream
Dash salt substitute
Dash black pepper

Combine all the ingredients in a blender, and blend until smooth. Chill 1 hour before serving. Top with fresh parsley and sprinkle with ground nutmeg.

Serves: 2

Cabbage Soup

2 cups shredded cabbage
2 cups cold water
2 teaspoons Smart Balance spread
2 tablespoons white onion, chopped
1 red bell pepper, chopped
1 teaspoon savory
1 teaspoon salt substitute

Place one teaspoon of the Smart Balance spread in a sauce pan, and put over low heat. Add the onion and sauté, until onion is tender. Add cabbage and bell pepper to skillet, cover and cook for 5 minutes stirring occasionally. Add water and savory and boil for 30 minutes. Add the other teaspoon of Smart Balance just before serving.

Serves: 2

Mushroom Soup

1 pound fresh mushrooms
1 medium white onion, sliced
5 cups cold water
1 parsley root, peeled and sliced
1 parsnip, peeled and sliced
1 small celery root, peeled and sliced
1 tablespoon Smart Balance spread
1 teaspoon salt substitute
1 tablespoon fresh parsley, chopped
¼ teaspoon ground black pepper

Peel the skin off the mushrooms, then wash and slice. Put the water in a sauce pan and bring to boil. Add onion, celery root, parsnip, and parsley root. Boil until vegetables are tender. Carefully place vegetable mixture in a blender. Cover and blend on medium speed for 3 minutes. Return mixture to the sauce pan. In a skillet sauté the mushrooms in ½ tablespoon Smart Balance spread. Add the mushrooms to the sauce pan and boil for 30 minutes. Add salt and the rest of the Smart Balance spread. Boil for additional 5 minutes. Garnish with parsley before serving.

Serve with 1 teaspoon fat-free sour cream (optional).

Serves: 3

Lentil Meatball Soup

½ pound lentils
2 quarts water
3 cups fat-free low-sodium chicken broth
2 teaspoons salt substitute
¼ teaspoon ground black pepper
1 white onion, chopped
2 celery stalks, chopped
1 parsley root, diced
1 red bell pepper, chopped
4 ripe tomatoes, chopped
½ pound 97% fat-free ground turkey
1 cup egg whites
½ baking soda
2 tablespoons fresh parsley, chopped

Rinse lentils. Put the water in a large sauce pan. Add the lentils and bring to boil. Add broth, onion, bell pepper, celery, parsley root, tomatoes, salt, and black pepper. Cover and simmer for one hour. Mix the ground turkey with egg whites, baking soda, and 1 tablespoon fresh parsley. Shape into small balls. Drop the meat balls into the soup. Simmer for 15 minutes, or until meat balls are fork-tender. Serve sprinkled with remaining of the fresh parsley.

Serves: 3

Black Eye Pea Soup

2 (15 ounces) cans black eye peas rinse and drained
1 cup chopped red bell pepper
1 cup chopped red onion
2 garlic cloves garlic, minced
1 cup chopped fresh tomatoes
1 dried chipotle pepper
1 tablespoon extra virgin olive oil
16 ounce fat-free low-sodium beef broth
2 tablespoons fresh parsley, chopped
1 teaspoon dried thyme
1 tablespoon fresh oregano, chopped

Cut the dry pepper open and discard seeds and stem. Cover pepper with boiling water for 30 minutes. Drain and cut pepper in small pieces. In a large sauce pan, put 1 tablespoon olive oil and place over medium heat. Cook the onion, garlic and red bell pepper for 3 minutes. Stir in dried pepper pieces, black eye peas, broth, tomato, parsley, thyme, and oregano. Bring to a boil. Reduce heat, cover and simmer for 30 minutes.
Before serving, garnish with fat-free sour cream and fresh parsley chopped (optional).

Serves: 2

Cauliflower Medley

2 tablespoons olive oil
2 cups fresh cauliflower florets
1 (10 ounces) package, frozen snow peas, thawed
1 garlic clove, minced
½ teaspoon salt substitute
Dash black pepper
2 tablespoon chopped pimiento

Heat the oil in skillet. Add garlic and cauliflower flowerets, and cook over low heat for 10 to 15 minutes, stirring occasionally. Add snow peas, salt, and pepper. Cover and cook 10 minutes longer. Stir in pimiento.

Serves: 3

Bean Medley

1(9 ounces) package, frozen French style green beans
1(9 ounces) package, frozen green beans
1(9 ounces) package frozen snow peas
2 tablespoons scallions, finely chopped
2 garlic cloves, minced
1 teaspoon Dijon mustard
3 tablespoons lemon juice
2 hard-cooked eggs
1 cup balsamic vinegar
Dash salt substitute
Dash black pepper

Cook vegetables according to package directions, and drain. Mix the scallions, garlic, mustard, lemon juice, balsamic vinegar, salt, and black pepper. Pour the sauce over the beans, and sprinkle the eggs on top.

Serves: 8

Oriental Celery

8 celery branches, sliced on the bias
1 cup fresh mushrooms, sliced
2 tablespoon Smart balance spread
¼ cup toasted almonds halves
Dash salt substitute
Dash black pepper

Cook celery in small amount of boiling water until just crisp-tender. Drain. Heat a skillet, and melt 2 tablespoons Smart Balance spread. Add the mushrooms and cook until tender. Add celery and almonds and toss lightly.

Serves: 2

Sauerkraut Delight

1(14 ounces) can sauerkraut
½ cup chopped white onion
½ cup low-sodium vegetable broth
2 tablespoons sesame seeds
½ cup fat-free sour cream
Dash black pepper

Rinse sauerkraut with cold water, and drain. Cook the onion in 3 tablespoons vegetable broth, on low heat, until tender. Add sauerkraut, broth, sesame seeds and pepper and mix lightly. Simmer covered for 10 to 12 minutes. Top with sour cream before serving.

Serves: 2

Cheddar Squash Casserole

5 cups zucchini, sliced and cooked
½ cup egg whites stiffly beaten
½ cup egg substitute
1 cup fat-free sour cream
1 ½ cup 2% fat cheddar cheese shredded
3 tablespoons fat-free bacon bites
¼ cup low-carbohydrates bread crumbs

Mix egg substitute, sour cream and bread crumbs. Fold in the egg whites. Layer half of the zucchini, egg mixture, cheese, and bread crumbs in a baking dish. Sprinkle with bacon bites. Repeat layers in the same order. Bake at 375 degrees for 20 minutes.

Serves: 4

Italian Style Salad

½ medium Boston lettuces, torn into bite-size pieces
6 romaine leaves, torn into bite-size pieces
3 green onions, sliced
8 radishes, sliced
½ cup sliced Portobello mushrooms
½ cup raw zucchini, sliced
¼ cup crumbled blue cheese
Dash salt
Dash pepper
Olive oil vinaigrette (see recipe)
1 garlic clove

Rub a large salad bowl with the garlic. Combine lettuce, zucchini, radish, green onion, and mushrooms. Add salt and pepper, and toss lightly with the dressing. Sprinkle blue cheese over.

Serves: 4

Spinach Salad I

1 pound fresh spinach
4 medium green onions, sliced
2 tablespoons cholesterol free bacon bites
1 tablespoon fresh lemon juice
2 tablespoons white wine vinegar
1 hard-cooked egg, chopped
1 tablespoon fresh parsley, chopped
1 teaspoon olive oil
Dash salt
Dash black pepper

Wash spinach, discard stems, and pat dry. Tear into a bowl, into bite-sizes pieces. Mix onion, lemon juice, vinegar, salt, pepper, oil and bacon bites. Pour dressing over spinach and toss to coat.
Sprinkle with egg and parsley.

Serves: 2

Three - Bean Salad

1 can, cut green beans
1 can wax beans
1 can, green beans French-style
1 medium green bell pepper, chopped
3 green onions, chopped
1 garlic clove, minced
2 tablespoons olive oil
½ cup white wine vinegar
1 teaspoon salt substitute
¼ teaspoon black pepper

Rinse and drain beans. Combine the beans in a salad bowl, and add pepper and green onion. Combine rest of ingredients and pour over beans; toss. Chill for at least four hours. Before serving toss again to coat beans and drain.

Serves: 2

Molded Chicken Salad

2 tablespoons unflavored gelatin
1½ cups boiling water
1½ cups cold water
½ cup white wine vinegar
1 tablespoon fresh lemon juice
1 cup finely shredded cabbage
½ cup celery, chopped
1 red bell pepper, chopped
½ chicken breast, grilled and chopped
Dash salt substitute
Dash black pepper

Mix gelatin, salt and pepper. Add the boiling water and stir until gelatin dissolves. Add cold water, lemon juice, vinegar, and chill until partially set. Fold in the vegetables and chicken breast. Pour into molding cups. Chill until firm. Unmold and serve over romaine lettuce.

Serves: 2

Chicken Salad Stuffed Tomatoes

1 chicken breast, grilled and chopped
1cup celery, finely chopped
1 cup red bell pepper, chopped
1 green onion, chopped
1 clove garlic, minced
2 tablespoons light mayonnaise
1 tablespoon cilantro, chopped
1 tablespoon lemon juice
Dash salt substitute
Dash black pepper
3 medium ripe tomatoes

Cut tomatoes in cups (cut thin slice from top, and scoop out center). Mix mayonnaise, lemon juice, garlic, cilantro, salt, and pepper. Add green onion, celery, red bell pepper and chicken. Toss. Fill tomatoes cups with mixture. Sprinkle on top with fresh parsley chopped (optional).Chill for one hour before serving. Serve over romaine lettuce.

Serves: 3

Tuna Salad Stuffed Tomatoes

1 (8 ounce) can white water packed tuna
1 cup celery, finely chopped
½ cup green bell pepper, chopped
1 garlic clove, minced
1 tablespoon lemon juice
1 tablespoon cilantro, chopped
2 tablespoons light mayonnaise
Dash salt substitute
Dash black pepper
3 medium ripe tomatoes

Cut tomatoes in daisies (turn tomato stem end down and cut down not quite through in 5 wedges; scoop out some of the center). Mix mayonnaise, lemon juice, garlic, cilantro, salt, and pepper.
Add celery, green pepper, and tuna and toss well. Fill the tomatoes with mixture. Chill before serving for one hour. Serve over a lettuce bad.

Serves: 3

Cheese Stuffed Tomatoes

1 cup fat-free, small curd cottage cheese
1 cup fat-free Feta cheese, crumbled
2 green onions, finely chopped
1 cup red bell pepper, chopped
1 teaspoon fresh dill, finely chopped
Dash black pepper
1 tablespoon fat-free bacon bites
6 pitted black olives, sliced
3 medium ripe tomatoes

Cut tomatoes in fantan (turn tomato stem end down and cut down not quite through in five slices).

Mix well cottage cheese, Feta cheese, green onion and black pepper. Add dill and bacon bites; toss. Fill tomatoes with the cheese mixture. Top with black olives slices. Serve over romaine lettuce leaves.

Serves: 3

Chef's Salad

8 romaine leaves, torn into bite-sizes pieces
1 cup 98% fat free turkey breast, cubed
1 cup part-skim mozzarella cheese, cubed
1 hard boiled egg, sliced
2 tablespoons olive oil vinaigrette (see recipe)

Arrange leaves in a bowl. Add turkey breast, cheese and egg. Pour dressing over.

Serves: 1

Mr. Benny's Mozzarella Salad

1(8 ounces) fresh mozzarella, sliced
1 large ripe tomato, sliced
1 tablespoon fresh parsley, chopped
1 tablespoon olive oil
1 tablespoon white wine vinegar
Salt substitute and ground black pepper, according to taste

On a salad plate alternate tomatoes slices and mozzarella slices, starting with tomatoes. Sprinkle each tomato slice with salt substitute and black pepper. Mix olive oil and vinegar; pour the mixture over to coat all slices. Sprinkle on top with fresh parsley.

Serves: 1

Crab Cakes

1 sweet potato, peeled and shredded
1 (6 ounces) can crab meat, drained
1 teaspoon salt substitute
1 teaspoon ground black pepper
1 cup egg whites
1 tablespoon fresh parsley, chopped
¼ cup green onion, finely chopped

Mix all the ingredients together until well blended. Preheat oven at 400 degrees. Spray a cookie sheet with nonstick cooking spray. Take one full tablespoon of crab mixture, at the time, and place on cookie sheet forming a ball. Leave about one inch between crab balls. Bake for 25 minutes or until golden brown. Remove from the oven and let it cool for 5 minutes. Serve crab cakes over lettuce.

Serves: 3

Cauliflower Salad

1 medium cauliflower
2 medium ripe tomatoes, sliced
8 romaine lettuce leave, torn into bite-size pieces
1 garlic clove, minced
1 tablespoon fresh parsley, chopped
1 tablespoon olive oil
2 tablespoons white whine vinegar
1 teaspoon Dijon mustard
Dash salt substitute
Dash black pepper

Separate cauliflower into flowerets. Boil in salted water for 10 minutes (or steam). Drain.

Line a salad bowl with romaine lettuce leaves, and add the tomatoes on top. Place the cauliflower florets in the middle. Mix the next 7 ingredients and pour over the cauliflower in the bowl. Chill for 30 minutes before serving.

Serves: 2

Spinach Salad II

1 pound fresh spinach
1 hard boiled egg, sliced
1 tablespoon olive oil
1 tablespoon red wine vinegar
1 garlic clove, minced
Dash salt
Dash black pepper

Rinse spinach and remove stems. Soak in boiling salted water for 2 minutes. Drain, and torn into bite-size pieces, in a salad bowl. Mix olive oil, vinegar, garlic, salt and black pepper; pour mixture over spinach. Toss. Add egg slices on top, before serving.

Serves: 1

Mushroom Salad

1 pound fresh whole mushrooms
1 tablespoon olive oil
2 tablespoons white wine vinegar
1 tablespoon fresh parsley, chopped
Dash salt substitute
Dash black pepper

Peel skin and rinse mushrooms. Boil in salted water for 10 minutes. Drain and slice. Mix next 5 ingredients, and pour the sauce over mushrooms. Toss and chill for 30 minutes before serving.

Serves: 2

Cod Stew

1 medium red onion, sliced
1 parsnip, sliced
1 celery root, sliced
2 medium tomatoes on the vine, sliced
1 cup green beans
1 cup wax beans
1 garlic clove, minced
3 bay leaves
Dash salt
Dash black pepper
4 cod fillets

Spray a skillet, generously with cooking spray. Cook the onion until golden and tender. Add parsnip, celery root, and garlic. Cook the vegetables until tender. Add tomatoes, beans, bay leaves salt, and pepper. Cook for additional 30 minutes. Add cod fillets to the skillet, and bake in the oven for 20 minutes at 400 degrees.

Discard the bay leaves and chill before serving.

Serves: 2

Tuna Meat Balls

3 cans (6ounces) solid white tuna in water
½ green bell pepper, finely chopped
½ white onion, grated
1 cup egg substitute
½ teaspoon salt substitute
½ teaspoon ground black pepper
1 tablespoon fresh dill, chopped

Mix all the ingredients together. Wet your hands, and shape mixture into little balls, flatted on top and bottom. Spray a skillet with nonstick cooking spray, and heat over medium heat. Add fish balls to the skillet and fry on each side until golden brown, flipping once.

Serving suggestions: serve over romaine lettuce; with tomato salad; with red cabbage salad.

Serves: 3

Salmon Soufflé

2 pounds salmon fillet, boiled
2 tablespoon Smart Balance spread
1 tablespoon whole wheat flour
1 cup fat-free milk
1 cup egg substitute
1 cup egg whites, stiffen
1 tablespoon part-skim mozzarella cheese, shredded
½ teaspoon salt
¼ teaspoon black pepper

Cut boiled salmon in cubes. Spray a skillet with nonstick cooking spray and place over medium heat. Melt 1 tablespoon Smart Balance spread. Blend in the flour and add milk, all at once. Cook over medium heat, stirring, until mixture thickens and bubbles. Remove from heat. Add fish, salt, 1 tablespoon Smart Balance spread, and black pepper to mixture. Let it cool until warm. Add egg substitute, 1 tablespoon at time. Fold in egg the whites. Pour into a sprayed, with nonstick cooking spray, casserole. Sprinkle cheese on top, and bake at 350 degrees for 45 minutes.

Serves: 3

Romanian Style Sweet Potato Salad

1 medium sweet potato
1 medium red onion, thinly sliced
1 hard boiled egg, sliced
1 cup black olives
1 teaspoon olive oil
2 tablespoons white wine vinegar
1 teaspoon salt substitute
Dash black pepper

Boil sweet potato until fork tender. Cool, peel and slice into ¼ inch slices. Combine sweet potato slices, onion rings, egg, black olives, salt, oil, and vinegar in a salad bowl. Refrigerate for 1 hour. Toss slightly before serving.

Serves: 2

Eggplant and Bell Pepper Casserole

3 medium eggplants
2 pounds tomatoes, sliced
2 red onions, thinly sliced
6 green bell peppers, sliced
3 garlic cloves cut in half
1 tablespoon olive oil
1 tablespoon fresh dill, chopped
1 tablespoon fresh parsley, chopped
1 teaspoon salt substitute
½ teaspoon ground black pepper

Cut the eggplant in four lengthwise; blanch in salted water and drain. Line the bottom of 1 ½-qt. casserole with half of tomato slices. Add onion, eggplant and green bell pepper in this order. Add garlic, dill and parsley. Line on top the other half of tomatoes. Cover and cook over low heat for 15 minutes. Add 1 tablespoon of olive oil, and cook in oven at 350 degrees for 40 minutes.

Serves: 3

Shrimp Chowder

2 medium sweet potatoes
1 medium parsnip
1 large parsley root
2 pounds medium shrimp, cooked and chopped
4 oz. Smoked salmon
2 celery stalks
1 chili pepper, seeded and chopped
1 can (4 ounce) water chestnut, finely chopped
1 teaspoon salt substitute (or according to taste)
¼ teaspoon ground black pepper
5 cups fat-free vegetable broth
1 tablespoon fresh cilantro, chopped
1 tablespoon fresh parsley, chopped

Peel potatoes, parsnip and parsley root. Rinse, slice and boil together with celery until tender. Drain. Put vegetables in blender, add smoked salmon and blend until everything is mixed well. You should obtain a thick paste. In a large sauce pan mix the vegetables paste, vegetable broth and bring to a boil. Add chili pepper, salt, black pepper and boil over low heat for 15 minutes, stirring frequently. Add shrimp and water chestnuts, and boil over low heat for10 more minutes. When ready pull away from heat, add parsley and cilantro. Garnish with 1 tablespoon low-fat fried onions before serving.

Serves: 4

Savory Shrimp

1 pound large shrimp
1 orange zest
1 lemon zest
1 teaspoon fresh thyme, chopped
1 teaspoon fresh oregano, chopped
Juice from 1 large orange
Juice from 1 medium lemon
¼ teaspoon paprika
1 tablespoon olive oil
1 garlic clove, minced

In a large skillet heat the olive oil. Add all the ingredients, and bring to a boil over low heat. Add shrimp to skillet and cook until tender.
Serve warm or cold, over romaine lettuce, or 1 cup whole wheat boiled spaghetti.

Serves: 4

Cauliflower Salad II

1 medium cauliflower
1 large tomato
2 teaspoons olive oil
1 teaspoon red wine vinegar
1 teaspoon lemon juice
1 tablespoon fresh parsley, chopped
1 teaspoon salt substitute
¼ teaspoon ground black pepper
1 tablespoon cold water

Separate cauliflower into flowerets. Wash and boil in salted water for 10 minutes; drain and place in salad bowl. Cut the tomato in thin slices and place over cauliflower. Mix well olive oil, lemon juice, vinegar, water, salt, pepper, and parsley. Pour sauce over and toss to coat.

Serves: 2

Cauliflower Salad III

1 medium cauliflower
1 red bell pepper
1 tablespoon walnuts, minced
1 tablespoon fresh parsley, chopped
1 teaspoon salt substitute
1 teaspoon white wine vinegar
2 tablespoons cold water
Dash ground black pepper

Separate cauliflower into flowerets; boil in salted water for 10 minutes, and drain. Remove stems and seeds from bell pepper and cut in thin slices. Place cauliflower and bell pepper in a salad bowl. Mix well water, vinegar, salt, black pepper, and parsley. Pour sauce over and toss. Sprinkle walnuts on top before serving.

Serves: 2

Greek Salad

8 romaine lettuce leaves, torn into bite-size pieces
1 cucumber, peeled, seeded and sliced
10 grape tomatoes
½ red onion, finely sliced
10 pitted black olives, sliced
1 cup grilled chicken breast, chopped
½ cup fat-free Feta cheese, crumbled
½ tablespoon olive oil
1 tablespoon fresh lemon juice
Dash ground black pepper

Combine lettuce, chicken, tomatoes, cucumber, onion, black olives, and cheese in large bowl.
Whisk together lemon juice and oil. Pour sauce over salad and toss to coat.

Serves: 1

Turkey Burgers with Mushroom Salsa

2 cans (6 ounces) mushrooms rinse and drained
½ cup tomatoes, peeled, seeded and chopped
1 tablespoon diced green chilies, drained
1 tablespoon fresh cilantro, chopped
1 tablespoon white wine vinegar
1 teaspoon olive oil
3 tablespoons egg whites
2 garlic cloves, crushed
12 ounces 97% lean ground turkey

Combine mushrooms, tomatoes, chilies, cilantro, oil, and vinegar in a small bowl. Cover and refrigerate for 1 hour. Combine turkey, garlic and egg whites, blend well, and shape to form four ¾ inches thick patties. Place on broiler pan and broil 5 inches from heat for 5 minutes. Turn and broil 5 to 8 minutes longer or until juice runs clear. Spoon the mushroom salsa over patties. Serve over a bad of lettuce.

Serves: 2

Chicken Kebabs over Wild Rice

½ cup white dry wine
2 tablespoons lemon juice
1 tablespoon olive oil
2 garlic cloves, crushed
2 tablespoon fresh cilantro, chopped
½ teaspoon salt substitute
½ teaspoon fresh ground black pepper
2 chicken breasts, skinless, boneless
1 medium red onion
1 medium red bell pepper
1 medium green bell pepper
12 small mushrooms
2 medium zucchini
Wooden or metal skewers
Nonstick cooking spray
3 cups cooked wild rice

Combine wine, lemon juice, garlic, olive oil, cilantro, salt, and pepper in a large bowl. Cut chicken breast into 1-inch pieces. Add the chicken to the bowl, and toss well to coat. Cover and refrigerate for 1 hour. Cut all the vegetables into 1-inch pieces. Remove chicken from the bowl and save the marinade. Alternately thread the chicken and vegetables, on each skewer. Place on broiler rack coated with nonstick cooking spray and brush with marinade. Broil 6 inches from heat, turning and brushing frequently with marinade.
Serve over hot rice. Garnish with fresh parsley.

Serves: 3

Marinated Chicken Breast

4 boneless, skinless chicken breast halves
1 tablespoon fresh rosemary leaves, chopped
3 cloves garlic, minced
¼ teaspoon ground black pepper
¼ teaspoon cayenne pepper
1 tablespoon extra virgin olive oil
1 cup dry white wine
1 tablespoon balsamic vinegar

Combine all ingredients in a large bowl. Add the chicken breast, toss to coat, cover and refrigerate for 4 hours. Remove chicken breast from the marinade, and place on a broiler rack. Broil on each side until golden brown and juices run out clear.
Serve over romaine lettuce.

Serves: 4

Chicken Salad

8 romaine lettuce leaves, torn into bite-size pieces
1 green bell pepper, seeded and cut into strips
½ English cucumber, sliced
10 cherry tomatoes, halved
1 cup green onion, chopped
1 half boneless skinless chicken breast, grilled and chopped
½ tablespoon olive oil
1 tablespoon balsamic vinegar

Combine lettuce, bell pepper, cucumber, green onion and cherry tomatoes in a salad bowl. Add olive oil, balsamic vinegar and toss well to coat. Put the chicken breast on top.

Serves: 1

Crab Salad

4 romaine lettuce leaves, torn into bite-size pieces
1 cup radicchio, shredded
½ cup cucumber, chopped
½ cup radishes, chopped
1 can (6ounces) crab meat drained
1 cup cherry tomatoes, chopped
1 tablespoon fat-free feta cheese, crumbled
1 tablespoon olive oil
2 tablespoon fresh lemon juice
1 clove garlic, minced
¼ teaspoon ground black pepper

Arrange lettuce on a large serving platter. Arrange radicchio, cucumber, radishes, and tomatoes in rows over lettuce. Mix olive oil, lemon juice, garlic, and pepper; drizzle over salad. Sprinkle on top with feta cheese.

Serves: 1

Orange Roughy Taco

Tortilla Shells:

8 whole wheat tortillas, 10 inches diameter

Have an empty can about 15-16 ounces. Remove label and one end from can. Wash the can and dry thoroughly. Spray entire surface of the can with nonstick cooking spray. Spray tortilla on both sides with nonstick cooking spray. Place tortilla over can, open end facing down. Bake in oven at 400 degrees for 5 minutes. Cool and remove the can. Turn tortilla shell upside down. Repeat with remaining tortillas.

Filling:

2 pounds Orange Roughy, fresh or frozen
1 tablespoon olive oil
4 medium ripe tomatoes, finely sliced
1 tablespoon red wine vinegar
2 teaspoons salt substitute
2 pounds white onion, chopped
3 tablespoons tomato paste
8 garlic cloves, minced
3 tablespoons dry red wine
1 teaspoon savory, finely chopped
2 dry bay leaves
½ teaspoon black peppercorn

Thaw fish in cold water if frozen, cut in 2 inch pieces and pat dry with paper towel. Spray a skillet with nonstick cooking spray and place over medium heat. Add fish to the skillet and cook one side for 5 minutes. Remove fish from skillet. Add the onion to skillet, and cook over low heat until golden. Add minced garlic, wine, tomato paste, salt, black pepper, bay leaves, savory, and vinegar. Boil for 10 minute. Put the sauce in a rectangular pan. Add the fish to the pan, with the uncooked side down. Place tomato slices on top of the fish and cook in the oven at 400 degrees for 15 minutes or until nice and brown.
    Divide among tortilla shells.

Serves: 8

Fish Taco

1 pound fresh or frozen tuna steaks
4 garlic cloves, minced
2 tablespoons fresh lemon juice
1 tablespoon fresh lime juice
1 tablespoon fresh cilantro, chopped
½ cup finely chopped green onion
4 tablespoons light mayonnaise
2 cups fresh cabbage, shredded
4 (16 inch) low-carbohydrate, low-fat whole wheat tortilla

Thaw fish if frozen, rinse and pat dry. Place fish on the rack of a broiler pan, sprayed with nonstick cooking spray. Season fish with salt substitute, fresh ground black pepper and 2 garlic cloves minced. Spray on top with nonstick cooking spray and broil, 4 inches from the heat, for 5 minutes. Using a spatula turn the fish and broil for 7 more minutes or until fish flakes easily when tested with a fork. Cool fish and break into ½ inch chunks using a fork.

Meanwhile, in bowl mix together mayonnaise, green onions, remaining garlic, cilantro, lemon juice, and lime juice. To assemble tacos: spread 1 tablespoon of mayo mixture, just enough to cover the entire surface, on each tortilla; divide fish chunks and cabbage among tortillas. Fold tortillas in half over filling.

Serves: 4

Chicken Breast Taco

1 boneless skinless chicken breast cut in thin strips
1 cup green onions, finely chopped
2 garlic cloves, minced
1 ½ cup cherry tomatoes, chopped
1 can (4 ounce) mushrooms, rinse and drained
1 fresh Anaheim pepper, seeded and finely chopped
3 tablespoons fresh parsley, chopped
2 tablespoon lemon juice
1 ½ cup lettuce, shredded
4 (10 inch) low-carbohydrate, low-fat, whole wheat tortillas
2% fat four cheese mix, shredded

Spray a skillet with nonstick cooking spray, and place over medium heat. Add ½ cup green onion and 1 garlic clove to the skillet, and cook for 5 minutes or until onion is tender. Add chicken strips and continue to cook, stirring occasionally, for 10 minutes or until chicken is tender and golden brown. Set aside. Meanwhile, in a bowl stir together tomatoes, the remaining of green onions, 1 garlic clove, Anaheim pepper, lemon juice, mushrooms, parsley, ½ teaspoon salt substitute, and ½ teaspoon ground black pepper. Cover and chill for 30 minutes. Preheat oven at 350 degrees. Wrap tortillas tightly in foil, and heat in the oven for 10 minutes. To assemble tacos, place lettuce in center of each warm tortilla. Divide chicken strips and salsa among tortillas. Top with shredded cheese. Fold tortillas in half over filling.

Serves: 4

Celery and Black Olives

4 medium celery roots, peeled and thinly sliced
6 medium ripe tomatoes
6 medium cucumbers, peeled, seeded and sliced
4 medium red onions, sliced
3 tablespoons pitted black olives
2 tablespoons olive oil
1 tablespoon fresh parsley, chopped
1 teaspoon salt substitute
2 cups cold water

In large pan heat oil add the celery slices, and sauté over low heat until fork tender. Add onion, cucumbers, tomatoes, and water, and cook over low heat for 35-40 minutes. Add olives and cook for additional 10 minutes. Serve cold, sprinkle with fresh parsley before serving.

Serves: 3

Crab and Wild Rice

½ cup green onion, chopped
1 cup celery, thinly sliced
2 cups fresh tomato, chopped
1 tablespoon fresh basil, chopped
2 tablespoons fresh parsley, chopped
½ teaspoon dried oregano
2 cloves garlic, minced
1 cup cooked wild rice
2 packages (8 ounces) fresh or frozen crab meat

Mix everything except rice and crab meat in a large skillet. Boil over low heat for 30 minutes, stirring occasionally. Stir in crab meat and boil until crab is tender, about 10 minutes.
    Add rice, stir and cook for another 5 minutes.

Serves: 2

Brine Cod

2 pounds frozen cod
1 tablespoon olive oil
5 garlic cloves, minced
½ teaspoon savory, chopped
1 chili pepper, chopped
1 teaspoon salt substitute
4 cups water

Thaw fish; wash and drain with paper towels. Brush each side of the fish with olive oil, sprinkle with salt and let it stand for 15 minutes. Bring the water to boil, remove from heat and pour water in a large bowl. Add salt and chili pepper. Add the fish, and let it stand for 10 minutes. Mix well garlic with olive oil, savory and 2 tablespoons of water. Add garlic mixture to the bowl. Refrigerate for 2 hours. Serve cold.
Serving suggestions: serve over romaine lettuce, or with mashed spinach.

Serves: 4

Shrimp Dijon

8 romaine leaves, torn into bite-size pieces
1 pound large shrimp, raw
2 cups fresh mushrooms, sliced
¼ cup dry white wine
½ teaspoon Dijon mustard
1 tablespoon lemon juice
¼ teaspoon paprika
1 clove garlic, crushed
1 teaspoon fresh parsley, chopped

In a large skillet, mix garlic, wine, Dijon mustard, paprika, lemon juice and bring to boil. Add the shrimp and cook for 15 minutes on low heat or until shrimps are no longer translucent. Remove from heat and cool. Serve over romaine lettuce, and garnish with sliced mushrooms.

Serves: 2

Easy Chicken Salad

2 halves grilled chicken breast, thin sliced
½ cup green onion, chopped
1 medium zucchini, thin sliced
½ cup grape tomatoes, chopped
½ cup black olives, thick sliced
1 cup artichoke hearts, rinsed, drained and sliced
10 romaine lettuce leaves, torn into bite-size pieces
1 tablespoon olive oil
1 clove garlic, minced
1½ tablespoon red wine vinegar
½ teaspoon salt substitute
Dash black pepper

In a glass bowl, whisk together olive oil, garlic, vinegar, salt, and black pepper. Add chicken breast, onion, zucchini, black olives, and artichoke hearts. Toss well to coat. Cover and refrigerate for one hour before serving. Serve over romaine lettuce.

Serves: 2

Chicken Hamburger

2 pounds 97% lean ground chicken breast
1 tablespoon fat-free sour cream
1 medium onion, baked
1 egg white, stiffen
2 teaspoon salt substitute
1 teaspoon ground black pepper
2 cloves garlic, minced
1 teaspoon Worcestershire sauce
1 teaspoon baking soda

In a large bowl mix well all ingredients. Cover with plastic rap and refrigerate for ½ hour.

Shape meat into patties. Spray a skillet with nonstick cooking spray. Place patties in skillet, and cook over high heat for 4 minutes. Turn and cook on the other side for additional 4 minutes or until juice runs clear.

Serve over romaine lettuce, with tomato and red onion slices.

Serves: 6

Burgers Supreme

Who said that if you are a diabetic, you have to go without your favorite food? So, if you like burgers and fries, and you miss having them, this is the recipe that will allow you to treat yourself. I guarantee you that it is a lot better that the regular fast food.

Burgers:

1 pound extra lean ground turkey breast
1 handful fresh parsley, chopped
1 small white onion, grated
1 teaspoon salt substitute
¼ teaspoon ground black pepper
1 cup 2% fat mozzarella cheese, shredded
1 teaspoon Dijon mustard

Mix all ingredients. Divide meat equally and shape in four patties. Grill until golden brown, flipping once.

Sauce:

2 plum tomatoes roasted
6 garlic cloves, roasted
1 medium white onion, roasted
1 tablespoon light mayonnaise
2 tablespoon fresh parsley
¼ teaspoon hot sauce

Put all ingredients in a food processor, and mix until well blend.

To assemble burgers:

Light rye bread
Tomato slices
Fresh baby spinach
4 red onion rings

Put 1 tomato slice on half slice bread, put burger on top, and add baby spinach and 1 onion ring. Spoon sauces over the second half slice of bread, and place it on top.

Use the remaining of the sauce to dip the sweet potato fries (see recipe).

If you like Portobello mushrooms, use one large grilled Portobello mushroom, to top your burger instead of the second half slice bread.

Serves: 4

DINNERS

Garlic Eggplant

1 medium eggplant, sliced in ½ inch rounds
3 garlic cloves, minced
1 teaspoon olive oil
3 teaspoons white wine vinegar
Dash salt or according to taste

Place the eggplant rounds on a PAM sprayed cooking sheet, and grill on each side until golden brown, flipping once. Mix the olive oil and the minced garlic until becomes like a paste.

Add the vinegar, 2 table spoons of water and mix together. Place the grilled eggplants rounds into a casserole and pour the garlic mixture over. Toss well and chill for 1 hour before serving.
Serving suggestions: with grilled chicken breast, or grilled steak.

Serves: 2

Stuffed Eggplant

1 medium eggplant
½ pound 98 % fat-free ground turkey
1 medium white onion, finely chopped
1 medium green bell pepper, chopped
3 tablespoons crushed tomatoes
1 garlic clove, minced
Dash salt
Dash pepper
Fresh parsley chopped

Cut the eggplant in half length wise, and scoop out the inside to leave like 1 inch wall. Grill on a PAM sprayed cooking sheet on low until soft, approximately 15 minutes. Spray a skillet with

PAM, and place over medium heat. Add the onion and garlic and cook until golden brown. Add the turkey meat, green pepper, and cook thoroughly for about 30 minutes. Add the tomatoes and cook for an additional 10 minutes. Stuff each eggplant half with the mixture, and bake at 400 degrees for 10 minutes.

Garnish with parley. Serve with 1 tablespoon fat-free sour cream.

Serves: 2

Eggplant Moussaka

2 medium eggplants
2 garlic cloves, minced
1 pound 98% fat-free ground turkey
1 package fresh mushrooms, sliced
1 cup egg substitute
1 cup 2% fat mozzarella cheese, shredded
Dash salt or to taste
Dash black pepper
1 teaspoon olive oil
2 cups tomato sauce

Slice the eggplant crosswise into ¼ inch rounds. Cook on a PAM sprayed skillet over medium heat, on each side, until golden brown. Set aside. Add the olive oil and garlic to the skillet and cook the garlic until golden. Add the meat and cook covered for 30 minutes stirring frequently. Add tomato juice and cook for 5 minutes. Set aside. Add ½ cup egg substitute, salt, and pepper and incorporate well into the meat. Into an oven safe casserole put one layer of eggplant rounds, one layer of mushrooms, one layer of meat sauce, one layer of mozzarella cheese, another layer of eggplant rounds and mozzarella cheese on top. Pour over the remaining ½ cup of egg substitute and bake at 400 degrees for about 30 minutes.

Serves: 4

Stuffed Peppers

3 medium red bell peppers
1 medium white onion
½ pound 98% lean ground turkey
2 cloves garlic, minced
1 small green pepper, finely chopped
1 can (6 ounce) mushrooms, rinse and drained
1 cup tomato juice
2 teaspoons salt substitute
Dash black pepper
1 teaspoon fresh dill finely chopped

Remove tops and seeds from the red peppers, and steam for about 20 minutes or until tender.

Meanwhile heat a Pam sprayed skillet. Add garlic, onion, green pepper and cook over low heat for 10 minutes, or until tender. Add ground turkey and cook for 30 minutes covered, stirring frequently. Add mushrooms, salt, black pepper, dill, and tomato juice. Cook covered for additional 15 minutes. Fill peppers with meat mixture. Top with 1 teaspoon fat-free sour cream.

Serves: 3

Romanian Style Stuffed Peppers

4 medium red bell peppers
1 medium white onion
2 cloves garlic, minced
1 cup wild rice cooked
2 cups tomato juice - divided
2 teaspoons salt substitute
½ teaspoon ground black pepper
2 tablespoons fresh parsley, chopped
1 pound 98% lean ground turkey

Remove tops and seeds from the red bell peppers, rinse and pat dry. Spray a skillet with nonstick coking spray and place over medium heat. Add onion and garlic to the skillet, and cook for 5 minutes or until onion is golden brown.

Add 1 cup tomato juice and cook for additional 7 minutes stirring constantly. Remove from heat and cool for 5 minutes. In a large bowl put meat, salt, black pepper, parsley, and rice. Add onion and tomato juice mixture to the bowl. Mix well until well combined. Fill peppers with meat and rice mixture. Preheat oven at 350 degrees. Put peppers in a baking dish. Add the other cup of tomato juice and ½ cup cold water. Cover with foil and bake for 1 hour or until peppers are fork tender. Remove foil and cook for additional 5 minutes.

To serve top with 1 teaspoon fat-free sour cream and sprinkle with fresh parsley (optional).

Serves: 4

Cod and Cabbage Delight

1 medium cabbage, shredded
2 pounds cod fillets, fresh or frozen
1 tablespoon Smart Balance spread
1 cup dry white wine
2 bay leaves
1 teaspoon salt
¼ teaspoon black pepper
¼ teaspoon allspice

Thaw cod fillets if use frozen according to package direction. Spray a large skillet with nonstick cooking spray and place over medium heat. Add cabbage to the skillet and cook covered until tender, stirring frequently. Move cabbage into an oven proof casserole. Add wine, allspice, salt, pepper, and bay leaves. Arrange cod filets on top. Cover filets with Smart Balance spread, and cook in the oven at 350 degrees, for 45 minutes or until fish is golden brown.

Serves: 4

Savory Salmon

2 pounds salmon fillet
1 tablespoon olive oil
1 cup dry white wine
3 medium white onions, finely sliced
2 clove garlic, minced
2 bay leaves
5 whole black peppercorns
1 cup tomato juice
1 teaspoon salt substitute

Place salmon in an oven proof casserole. Add rest of the ingredients. Cook in the oven at 350 degrees for about 45 minute. Once in a while spread sauce over salmon.
Serving suggestions: serve with mashed sweet potatoes, mashed spinach, steamed vegetables.

Serves: 4

Orange Roughy Casserole

2 pounds Orange Roughy
2 cups fat-free, low-sodium, vegetable broth
2 pounds fresh mushrooms, thick sliced
1 tablespoon Smart Balance spread
½ tablespoon whole wheat flour
2 cloves garlic, crushed
1 cup fat-free sour cream
2 cups part-skim mozzarella cheese, shredded
Dash black pepper
2 basil leaves

Bring vegetable broth to a boil. Add the fish, and boil over low heat for 7 minutes. Remove fish, let it cool, and cut in cubes. Spray a skillet with nonstick cooking spray. Add mushrooms to skillet and cook over medium heat, stirring frequently until all moister is gone. Remove mushrooms and cool. In a pan, melt 1 tablespoon Smart Balance spread, and bland in the flour. Add sour cream and garlic all at once, and bring to a boil. Remove sauce from heat.

Spray an oven proof casserole with nonstick cooking spray. Place one layer of each: fish, mushrooms, sauce and cheese. Repeat in same order. Bake at 400 degrees for 15 minutes.

Serves: 4

Meat Balls in Tomato Sauce

2 pounds ground loin beef
2 scallions, finely chopped
1 celery stalk with leaves, finely chopped
1 clove garlic, crushed
4 ripe tomatoes, peel, seeded, and chopped
½ cup tomato juice
2 bay leaves
2 tablespoons fresh parsley, chopped
½ teaspoon salt substitute
¼ teaspoon black pepper
½ cup egg whites

Mix well ground beef, scallion, garlic, 1 tablespoon parsley, salt, black pepper, and egg whites.

Shape beef mixture into small balls. Spray a skillet with nonstick cooking spray, and place over medium heat. Add meat balls to the skillet and fry for 5 minutes on each side or until golden brown. Coat a sauce pan with nonstick cooking spray. Add tomatoes, tomato juice, celery, and bay leaves. Cook over medium heat stirring frequently for 15 minutes. Add meat balls to sauce and cook for additional 10 minutes. Add 1 tablespoon parsley and remove from heat.

Serves: 6

Cabbage Casserole

1 medium cabbage
2 ½ pounds 98% fat-free ground turkey
1 medium red onion, chopped
1 teaspoon salt substitute
¼ teaspoon thyme
¼ teaspoon black pepper
3 tablespoon fat-free sour cream

Spray a skillet with nonstick cooking spray. Add onion, cover and cook for 5 minutes. Add meat, salt, pepper, and thyme. Cover and cook for 15 minutes stirring frequently.

Blanch the cabbage, drain, and cool till easy to maneuver. Separate leaves. Spray a baking pan with nonstick cooking spray. Put the cabbage and the meat in the pan, alternating layers of cabbage leaves and meat. Last layer should be cabbage. Spread the sour cream on top. Cook for 35 minutes at 350 degrees or until cabbage is fork tender.

Serves: 4

Cauliflower Casserole

1 big cauliflower
2 pounds 98% fat-free ground chicken
1 medium white onion, chopped
1 tablespoon Smart Balance spread
1 egg
2 tablespoons light rye bread crumbs
1 teaspoon salt substitute
¼ teaspoon black pepper
1 clove garlic, minced

Boil cauliflower flowerets in salted water for 10 minutes. Drain and cool. Spray a skillet with nonstick cooking spray. Add onion and garlic to the skillet, cover and cook for 2 minutes over low heat. Add meat, salt, and peeper continue to cook, stirring frequently for 20 minutes.

Coat a baking pan with Smart Balance spread and bread crumbs. Place one layer of cauliflower flowerets, one layer of meat and another layer of cauliflower flowerets. Sprinkle 1 tablespoon bread crumbs on top. Beat the egg with 2 tablespoons of water; pour mixture over on top.

Bake at 350 degrees for 40 minutes.

Serves: 4

Meat Loaf

1 pound 97% fat free ground turkey
1 medium white onion, grated
1 garlic clove, minced
1 tablespoon fresh parsley, chopped
1 tablespoon fat-free sour cream
1 teaspoon salt substitute
1 teaspoon black pepper
2 tablespoons sesame seeds
3 tablespoon egg whites
2 tablespoons egg substitute

Combine ground turkey, onion, garlic, parsley, sour cream, salt, pepper, and egg substitute.

Mix well. Shape it like a roll. Mix egg whites and sesame seeds. Coat meat roll with egg mixture. Spray a pan with nonstick cooking spray. Place the meat roll in the pan and bake at 375 degrees for 45 minutes. Slice before serving.

Serving suggestions: with toss salad, mashed sweet potatoes and red bell pepper salad, tomato salad, cucumber salad

Serves: 3

Tuna Rolls

1 boneless, skinless chicken breast
2 cans chunk tuna in water
2 tablespoons fresh parsley, chopped
1 cup low-fat, low-sodium, vegetable broth
1 teaspoon salt substitute
1 teaspoon black pepper
1 garlic clove, minced
½ cup dry white wine

Slice chicken breast lengthwise into ½ inch pieces, and pound to ¼ inch thick. Drain tuna and mix together with parsley, garlic, salt, and pepper. Place 1 tablespoon of mixture, in the middle of the flatten chicken breast. Roll up and fasten edges with skewers. Grill 5 inches from the top for 5minutes, turning once.

Spray a baking pan with nonstick cooking spray. Place rolls in baking pan, add vegetable broth, and wine. Bake for 30 minutes at 375 degrees. Baste from time to time.

Serves: 2

Dijon Steak

1 pound sirloin steak 1 inch thick
1 tablespoon Dijon mustard
1 cup low-fat, low-sodium, beef broth
½ pound mushrooms, sliced
1 medium red onion, thin sliced
1 tablespoon Smart Balance spread
1 cup dry red wine
1 garlic clove, minced

Grill steak 5 inch from top for 5 minutes on each side. Coat the steak with mustard. Spray a baking pan with nonstick cooking spray. Place the steak in the pan, and pour the beef broth over. Bake at 350 degrees for 20 minutes. Meanwhile place the spread in a frying pan. Add mushrooms, onion and garlic. Cook for 5 minutes on low heat. Add wine, and cook for additional 10 minutes. Pour sauce over steak and bake for additional 10 minutes.

Serves: 2

Roasted Salmon

1 salmon fillet
1 tablespoon olive oil
1 parsley root, peeled and finely sliced
1 small celery root, peeled and finely sliced
1 carrot, peeled and finely sliced
2 medium red onions, finely sliced
½ teaspoon ground black pepper
1 teaspoon salt substitute
3 tablespoons cold water

Wash salmon and cut in 5 inch pieces. Drain with paper towel. Spray a rectangular pan with nonstick cooking spray. Put all vegetables in layers in the pan. Put salmon pieces on top. Add salt, black pepper, oil, and water. Cook in oven at 375 degrees for 40 minutes. Baste fish with pan juice, and turn to cook on other side. Continue to cook for additional 10 minutes or until fish is golden brown.

Serves: 4

Marinated Mahi-Mahi

2 pounds Mahi-Mahi fish, fresh or frozen
2 tablespoons olive oil

Sauce:
3 bay leaves
1 medium red onion
½ teaspoon black peppercorn
2 tablespoons tomato paste
1 chili pepper
1 teaspoon salt substitute
5 cups cold water
1 tablespoon soy flour

Wash fish and drain (if frozen thaw in cold water). Spray a skillet with nonstick cooking spray and place over medium heat. Add fish to the skillet and cook on each side until golden, flipping once. In a sauce pan add water and bring to a boil. Add black peppercorn, onion finely sliced and bay leaves. Boil for 5 minutes. Add tomato paste, salt, soy flour, and chili pepper. Boil until sauce thickens. Add fish to sauce and boil for 10 minutes. Serve cold.

Serves: 3

Romanian Style Baked Salmon

1 salmon fillet (about 2 pounds)
2 medium white onions, chopped
3 tablespoons pitted black olives
1 tablespoon olive oil
1 teaspoon savory, chopped
1 teaspoon tomato paste
1 small pickle, sliced
½ pound fresh mushrooms, peeled, washed and chopped
1 cup dry white wine
1 fresh lemon
1 tablespoon fresh parsley, chopped
1 teaspoon salt substitute
½ teaspoon ground black pepper

Spray a large skillet with nonstick cooking spray. Add onion to skillet and cook until onion is translucent. In a rectangular pan put the cooked onion, mushrooms, pickle, and olives. Mix tomato paste and wine, and pour the sauce over in pan. Add salmon cut in 4 inch pieces. Add savory, salt and black pepper. Baste fish with sauce and cook in oven at 375 degrees for 20 minutes. Baste from time to time.

Serve cold. Sprinkle with fresh parsley before serving and garnish with lemon slices.

Serves: 4

Boiled Cod

2 pounds cod fillet, fresh or frozen
1 large carrot
2 parsley roots
1 celery root
3 medium red onions, sliced
1 teaspoon black peppercorn
2 bay leaves, dry
2 tablespoons fresh lemon juice
3 tablespoons dry white wine
1 tablespoon fresh parsley, chopped
2 tablespoons white wine vinegar
4 garlic cloves, minced
1 teaspoon salt substitute

Peel skin off carrot, parsley roots and celery. Wash and cut in ½ inch slices. Put vegetables in a large sauce pan. Add water just to cover the vegetables, and bring to boil. Add onion and boil until vegetables are fork tender. Add rest of ingredients. Add fish cover and boil over low heat for 10 minutes or until fish is fork tender (do not over boil).

Serve at once.

Serves: 4

Spaghetti Squash

2 pounds spaghetti squash, halved lengthwise and seeded
1 pound 98% lean ground turkey
1 red onion, chopped
1 celery stalk, chopped
1 small green bell pepper, thin sliced
1 cup fresh mushrooms, sliced
2 plum tomatoes, diced
½ teaspoon salt substitute
½ teaspoon ground black pepper
1 cup low-sugar tomato juice
½ cup low-fat Parmesan cheese, grated
1 tablespoon fresh parsley, chopped
3 cloves garlic, chopped

Place the squash halves, cut side down in a microwave safe dish. Add ½ cup water, cover with plastic wrap and microwave on high for 10 minutes, or until tender. Drain and cool slightly.

Meanwhile, spray generously a large skillet with nonstick cooking spray and place over medium heat. Add onion and garlic to the skillet, and cook for 3 minutes or until onion is translucent. Add green pepper and mushrooms and cook for additional 5 minutes. Add the meat and cook for 15 minutes stirring occasionally or until meat is nice and brown. Add tomatoes, salt, black pepper, and tomato juice. Reduce heat, cover and simmer for 15 minutes.

Using a fork, scrape the squash strands into a large bowl. Pour meat sauce over the squash. Sprinkle Parmesan cheese on top. Garnish with parsley.

Serves: 4

Chicken Supreme

4 skinless, boneless chicken breast halves
6 ripe tomatoes, seeded and sliced
½ cup green bell pepper, chopped
½ cup red bell pepper, chopped
1 can water chestnut, rinse and drained
3 clove garlic, crushed

2 tablespoons lemon juice
1 teaspoon lemon peel
½ cup tomato juice
1 tablespoon fresh cilantro, chopped
1 teaspoon salt substitute
¼ teaspoon black pepper
¼ teaspoon thyme

Spray a large skillet with nonstick cooking spray. Add garlic, onion and 1 tablespoon lemon juice; cover and cook for 5 minutes. Add tomatoes, green pepper, red pepper, water chestnut, 1 tablespoon lemon juice, lemon peel, cilantro, thyme, and tomato juice to the skillet and stir to mix. Cook over medium heat, stirring frequently for 10 minutes. Rub salt and pepper into the chicken breast. Place chicken over tomato mixture. Reduce heat to low, cover and cook stirring and turning frequently for 15 minutes.

Arrange chicken on serving plate and spoon sauce over chicken.

Serves: 4

Rosemary Chicken Delight

4 skinless, boneless chicken breast halves
¼ cup dry vermouth
1 tablespoon fresh rosemary, finely chopped
3 cloves garlic, crushed
1 tablespoon olive oil
1 teaspoon light soy sauce
1 tablespoon fresh lemon juice
¼ teaspoon ground black pepper

Combine vermouth, rosemary, garlic, olive oil, soy sauce, lemon juice, and black pepper in a shallow glass dish. Add chicken breast, turning to coat. Cover and refrigerate for 2 hours. Spray a broiler pan with nonstick cooking spray. Remove chicken from marinade. Broil 6 inch form heat until golden brown. Turn on the other side and brush with marinade. Broil until golden brown or till juice runs out clear.

Serves: 4

Chicken Chili

1 skinless boneless chicken breast, chopped
1 celery stalk, chopped
1 red onion, chopped
4 garlic cloves, minced
1 green bell pepper, chopped
1 red bell pepper, chopped
1 can (15 ounces) kidney beans rinse and drained
1 can (15 ounces) garbanzo beans rinse and drained
1 teaspoon dried oregano
1 teaspoon chili powder
¼ teaspoon crushed red pepper flakes
1 cup cherry tomatoes, chopped
1½ cup low-sugar tomato juice
1 teaspoon dry savory
1 tablespoon fresh parsley, chopped
1 cup 2% fat shredded Cheddar cheese

Spray a large sauce pan with nonstick cooking spray. Place over medium heat. Add onion and garlic to the pan. Cook stirring constantly until onion is translucent. Add chicken to the pan, and cook until chicken is golden brawn. Add rest of ingredients and stir. Cook over low heat for 30 minutes, until sauce thickens. Pull away from heat. Sprinkle on top with fresh parsley.

Sprinkle on top with shredded cheese before serving.

Serves: 2

Beef and Mushrooms Delight

2 pounds top sirloin beef
1 cup fat-free, low-sodium, vegetable broth
1 pound fresh mushrooms, sliced
½ tablespoon whole wheat flour
½ cup green onion, chopped
1 cup dry white wine
3 tablespoons fat-free sour cream
1 teaspoon salt substitute

¼ teaspoon black pepper
1 clove garlic, crushed

Rub in the beef steak ½ teaspoon salt and garlic. Spray a broiling pan with nonstick cooking spray; place steaks on broiling pan and broil 5 inch from heat for 5 minutes on each side. Set aside and cool till easy to handle, than cut into 1 inch slices. Spray a skillet with nonstick cooking spray. Add mushrooms, green onion and sauté over low heat for 5 minutes. Add flour to skillet, and mix frequently until well blended. Add wine and vegetable broth, and boil for 5 minute or until sauce thickens.
Place meat slices in an oven proofed casserole, and coat with mushrooms sauce. Cover and cook in oven at 400 degrees for 30 minutes. Add sour cream and cook for 5 more minutes.

Serves: 4

Chicken and Celery Casserole

1 whole boneless, skinless chicken breast, sliced
1 large celery root, ¼ inch thick sliced
1 medium red onion, sliced
2 garlic cloves, minced
1 cup tomato juice
1 tablespoon fresh parsley, chopped
1 teaspoon salt substitute
¼ teaspoon black pepper
2 bay leaves

Spray a skillet with nonstick cooking spray. Add onion, garlic, meat, salt, pepper, and ¼ cup water; cover and sauté over low heat for 15 minutes. Remove from heat, and place the meat mixture into an oven proof casserole. Add celery, tomato juice, bay leaves, and parsley. Cook in oven for 30 minutes at 375 degrees.

Serves: 2

Beef Stew

1 pound lean beef meat cut in 1½ inch strips
½ medium cabbage, chopped
1 parsley root, sliced
½ celery root, sliced
1 cup green beans
1 cup waxed beans
1 cup okra
1 medium zucchini, thick sliced
1 medium eggplant, thick sliced
1 cup cauliflower flowerets
3 medium ripe tomatoes cut in half
1 green bell pepper, chopped
1 teaspoon salt substitute
¼ teaspoon black pepper
1 tablespoon chives, chopped
1 clove garlic, minced
1 scallion, chopped
1 cup low-sugar, tomato juice
1 cup water

In a large sauce pan, sauté the onion, garlic, and meat, for 10 minutes over low heat. Add parsley and celery to the pan, cover and sauté for ten minutes. Add rest of the ingredients. Cover and simmer for 30 minutes, or until meat and vegetables are fork-tender.

Serves: 3

Cauliflower Chicken

1 skinless, boneless chicken breast
1 medium cauliflower
1 medium white onion, finely chopped
1 tablespoon Smart Balance spread
2 tablespoons fat-free sour cream
1 clove garlic, minced
2 teaspoons salt substitute

½ teaspoon black pepper
1 cup low-fat, low-sodium vegetable broth
1 tablespoon fresh parsley, chopped

In a sauce pan heat the Smart Balance spread and garlic. Add onion, and chicken breast, and sauté quickly over medium heat until brown. Set aside. Meanwhile blanch cauliflower flowerets. Drain and add them to the chicken. Mix well vegetable broth, sour cream, parsley, salt, and pepper. Pour mixture over chicken and cauliflower. Cover and boil over low heat for 15 minutes.

Serves: 2

Chicken Hamburger

2 pounds 97% lean ground chicken breast
1 tablespoon fat-free sour cream
1 medium onion, baked
1 egg white, stiffen
2 teaspoon salt substitute
1 teaspoon ground black pepper
2 cloves garlic, minced
1 teaspoon Worcestershire sauce
1 teaspoon baking soda

In a large bowl mix well all ingredients. Cover with plastic rap and refrigerate for ½ hour.

Shape meat into patties. Spray a skillet with nonstick cooking spray. Place patties in skillet and cook over high heat for 4 minutes. Turn and cook on the other side for additional 4 minutes or until juices runs clear.
Serving suggestions: Serve over romaine lettuce, with tomato and red onion slices.

Serves: 4

Hawaiian Style Chicken Breast

2 cups crushed unsweetened pineapple
2 medium sweet potatoes, pared and sliced
3 boneless skinless chicken breasts
¼ teaspoon salt substitute
¼ teaspoon ground black pepper
¼ teaspoon paprika
3 turkey bacon strips

Preheat oven to 350 degrees. Place pineapple in a large baking dish. Add paprika and toss. Put potato slices on top of pineapple. Season the chicken breast with salt, and pepper. Place chicken breast on top of sweet potatoes. Place one bacon strip on top of each chicken breast. Cover and bake for 45 minutes or until chicken breast is tender. Remove cover, and increase the oven temperature to 450 degrees. Cook for 10 more minutes until chicken breast is golden brown.

Serves: 6

Chicken Stir and Fry

1 pound boneless skinless chicken breast cut crosswise, in strips
¾ cup fat-free, low-sodium, chicken broth
¼ cup light teriyaki sauce
1 tablespoon light sesame oil
2 tablespoons garlic, chopped
2 tablespoons fresh ginger, grated
2 tablespoons extra-virgin olive oil
½ pound fresh broccoli
½ pound snow peas
1 red bell pepper cut in ½ inch wide, strips
6 scallions, coarsely chopped

Heat 1 tablespoon olive oil, in a large nonstick skillet over medium heat, until hot. Add chicken strips and stir-fry 5 minutes or until lightly browned and cooked through. Remove to a platter. In a small bowl, make the sauce, by stirring chicken broth, teriyaki sauce, sesame oil, garlic, and ginger, until blend. Heat remaining 1 tablespoon olive oil in the skillet. Add scallions, broccoli, snow peas, and red pepper. Stir-fry for 6 minutes or until tender. Add sauce to the skillet and cook for 2 minutes. Stir in chicken strips and heat through.

Serves: 3

Stuffed Orange Roughy

6 Orange Roughy fillets
1 small white onion, chopped
1 can (3 ounces) chopped mushrooms, drained
1 can crab meat, drained and flaked
¼ cup wheat germ
2 tablespoons fresh parsley, chopped
½ teaspoon salt substitute
1 tablespoon Smart Balance spread
2 tablespoon soy flour
1 cup 2% fat milk
½ teaspoon ground black pepper
½ cup dry white wine
1 tablespoon fresh lemon juice
1 garlic clove, minced
1 cup part-skim mozzarella cheese, shredded

Spray a skillet with nonstick cooking spray, and place over low heat. Add the onion, cover and cook until translucent. Set aside. Stir in mushrooms, crab meat, wheat germ, parsley, salt, and black pepper. Spread mixture over fillets, roll and place seam down, in a baking dish. In a sauce pan melt Smart Balance spread and blend in the flour. Stir in milk and wine. Add lemon juice and garlic. Cook and stir until mixture thickens. Pour the sauce, over rolled fillets. Bake in oven at 400 degrees for 25 minutes. Sprinkle with cheese, return to oven, and bake for 5 more minutes.

Serves: 6

Beef Rolls

1 pound extra lean ground beef
1½ cup tomato sauce
½ teaspoon salt substitute
½ teaspoon ground black pepper
1 cup part-skim ricotta cheese
½ cup 2% fat, mild cedar cheese, shredded
1 cup egg whites
2 tablespoons fresh parsley, chopped
2 garlic cloves, minced
1 teaspoon dry savory

Mix ground beef, ¼ cup tomato juice, savory, salt and black pepper. Shape into 9x12 inch rectangle, on a sprayed foil. Mix ricotta cheese, egg whites, cedar cheese, garlic and fresh parsley. Spread on ground beef. Roll like a jelly roll using foil to shape. Shape foil around loaf leaving top exposed. Pour remainder of tomato juice over meat roll. Bake at 350 degrees for 35 minutes.

Serves: 4

Chicken and Tomatillo Stew

2 pounds tomatillo, husked, rinsed and halved
4 Serrano peppers, stemmed and seeded
1 white onion, quartered
3 cloves garlic, peeled
1 cup fat-free, low-sodium, chicken broth
¼ teaspoon dried caraway
2 pounds boneless skinless chicken breast cut in 1½ inch cubes
2 tablespoon fresh parsley, chopped
1 cup fat-free Feta cheese, crumbled
Salt and black pepper to taste

Preheat the broiler. Place tomatillo, peppers, onion, and garlic on a baking sheet. Broil for 5 to 8 minutes, turning occasionally. Remove from broiler and cool. Put vegetables in a food processor. Add chicken broth and caraway. Process the vegetables until smooth.

Place chicken breast cubes on a baking sheet. Broil for 5 minutes on each side. Remove from broiler. In a sauce pan, transfer chicken cubes, and pour the sauce, from the food processor, over. Add parsley, salt, and pepper. Bring to a boil. Reduce heat, cover and simmer for 1 hour.

Before serving sprinkle each serving with feta cheese.

Serves: 4

Romanian Style Stuffed Zucchini

6 zucchini 8" long
¾ ponds 97% fat-free ground turkey
1 small onion, finely chopped
2 teaspoons salt substitute
½ teaspoon ground black pepper
2 tablespoons fresh parsley, chopped
1 cup whiled rice, cooked
2 tablespoon tomato paste

Peel zucchini. Cut off the end, wash, drain and core out the centers. Spray a skillet with nonstick cooking spray. Place over low heat, add onion and cook until translucent. Add 1 tablespoon tomato paste and cook for 5 minutes stirring constantly. In a bowl mix meat, rice, salt, pepper, and parsley. Add onion and mix well. Stuff the mixture into cored zucchini. Place stuffed zucchini in a rectangular, sprayed with nonstick cooking spray, baking pan. Dissolve 1 tablespoon tomato paste in 1cup water. Pour over stuffed zucchini. Cook in oven at 350 degrees for 1 hour or until zucchini are fork tender. Flip the zucchini over, on the other side, half way through.

Serves: 3

Grilled Tuna Steak with Salsa

Salsa:
2 cups grape tomatoes cut in halves
½ cup white onion, chopped
1 Pasilla (Chile Negro) pepper, seeded and finely chopped
1 cup fresh cranberries
2 garlic cloves, minced
1 teaspoon fresh rosemary, chopped
1 tablespoon fresh parsley, chopped
2 tablespoons apple-cider vinegar
1 tablespoon extra-light virgin olive oil
Salt substitute and ground black pepper to taste

Put all ingredients in a bowl. Toss to coat. Cover and refrigerate for two hours before serving.

Tuna:
2 tuna steaks (about half pound each)
Salt and pepper to taste

Heat the grill for searing. Season the tuna steaks, on both sides, with salt and pepper. Sear tuna on both sides until browned and cooked to desire doneness.

To serve, line a platter with fresh arugula. Place tuna next to salad. Spoon the salsa over tuna steak. Garnish with fresh rosemary sprigs.

Serves: 2

Steak and Sweet Potato Casserole

1 pound loin steak
2 medium sweet potatoes
1 red onion, finely sliced
1 tablespoon olive oil
1 teaspoon salt substitute
1 teaspoon ground black pepper
2 tablespoons fresh parsley, chopped

2 cups tomato sauce
2 garlic cloves, minced

Cut steak into 2 inch pieces. Rub in salt and pepper on each side. Grill on high until brown on each side. Place meat in a rectangular pan. Peel potatoes, rinse, and cut in fourths. Arrange potatoes with meat. Sprinkle onion, garlic, salt, pepper, and parsley over all. Add tomato sauce, cover and cook in the oven for 30 minutes. Uncover and cook for additional 10 minutes. Do not overcook potatoes.

Serves: 4

Stuffed Chicken Breast

6 skinless, boneless chicken breasts
4 green onions, chopped
1 small red bell pepper, finely chopped
1 can (6 ounces) mushrooms, rinsed, drained and chopped
2 tablespoons fresh parsley, chopped
1 tablespoon olive oil
½ cup dry white wine
4 garlic cloves, minced
2 tablespoons egg whites
Salt substitute and ground black pepper to taste
1 teaspoon balsamic vinegar

Quickly pound out chicken breast with mallet or rolling pin to flatten. Spray a skillet with nonstick cooking spray and place over low heat. Add onion, bell pepper, and sauté until tender. When ready mix with mushrooms, parsley, egg whites, salt, and pepper. Brush each chicken breast with balsamic vinegar. Spread one tablespoon or so, of mixture evenly on each chicken breast. Roll up and place seam-side down in a baking dish. Roast at 400 degrees for 15 to 20 minutes. Mix olive oil, wine and garlic. Pour sauce over chicken breast and continue cooking for10 to 15 minutes. To check that chicken is cook through, cut carefully into center of one roll with tip of sharp knife. Serve in slices, warm.

Serves: 12

Stuffed Chicken Breast and Wild Rice

4 large boneless, skinless chicken breast halves
2 tablespoons garlic, minced
2 cans (6 ounces) crab meat, drained and flaked
8 ounces 2% fat mild cheddar cheese, shredded
3 tablespoons fresh parsley, finely chopped
½ cup egg substitute
1 cup rye bread crumbs
1 cup dry white wine
2 cups boiled wild rice
1 cup fat-free, low-sodium, chicken broth
¼ teaspoon cayenne pepper

Flatten chicken to ¼ inch thickness. Spread 1 teaspoon garlic on one side of each chicken breast half. Place crab meat, cheese, and parsley down the center of each. Roll up and tuck in ends; secure with toothpicks. In a bowl, beat egg substitute and cold water. Place bread crumbs and cayenne pepper in another bowl, and mix. Dip chicken in egg mixture then roll in bread crumbs.

Spray a skillet with nonstick cooking spray. Brown the chicken breasts on both sides.

Transfer chicken to a baking dish. Add dry wine and chicken broth. Bake uncovered at 375 degrees for 30 minutes or until chicken juices run clear. Serve over wild rice.Garnish with fresh parsley.

Serves: 4

Stuffed Acorn Squash

1 boneless, skinless chicken breast, grilled and chopped
1 cup wild rice
2 cups fat-free, low-sodium, vegetable broth
½ teaspoon dried thyme
1 cup celery, finely chopped
1 medium red onion, chopped
1 tablespoon olive oil
¼ cup almonds, toasted and coarsely chopped
1 tablespoon fresh parsley, chopped
2 medium acorn squash
Ground black pepper to taste
2 cloves garlic, minced

In a large sauce pan, sauté onion, garlic and celery until tender. Stir in wild rice and vegetable broth. Bring to a boil. Reduce heat, cover and simmer for 35 minutes or until rice is tender and liquid is almost absorbed. Remove from heat. Stir in chicken breast, thyme, almonds, black pepper and parsley.

Cut squash in half width wise. Remove and discard seeds and membranes. With a sharp knife, cut a thin slice from the bottom of each half, so squash sits flat. Fill squash halves with rice-chicken mixture. Place in a baking pan. Add 1 cup water to the pan. Spray a heavy duty foil with nonstick cooking spray. Cover pan tightly with foil, coated side down. Bake, at 375 degrees for 50 minutes or until squash is tender. Garnish with fresh parsley before serving.

Serves: 4

Turkey Breast with Spicy Sauce

2 turkey breast, tenderloins
1 white onion cut in rounds
1 cup celery, sliced
3 cups fat-free, low-sodium, chicken broth
2 parsnip roots
1 large sweet potato
3 cups water

Season the turkey breast, with salt substitute, and fresh ground black pepper. Spray a large pan with nonstick cooking spray, and place over medium heat. Add meat to pan, and sear until brown on each side. Add onion and celery, and cook for five minutes. Add broth and water, cover and simmer for 45 minutes. Peel parsnip, rinse and slice. Peel sweet potato, rinse and cut in thick slices. Add parsnip and potato to the pan. Simmer for another 40 minutes or until parsnip and potato is fork tender.

Sauce:
2 shallots, chopped
4 cloves garlic, chopped
1 teaspoon capers
¼ teaspoon red pepper flakes
1 tablespoon extra-virgin olive oil, cold press
Salt and ground black pepper to taste
2 tablespoons fresh parsley, chopped

Mix all ingredients until well combined in a bowl.

To serve: Slice turkey breast. Put turkey on a serving platter on one side and vegetables on the other side of platter. Pour sauce over turkey, and garnish with fresh parsley sprigs.

Serves: 3

SNACKS

Remember, snacks will help you feel full; avoid hunger, and the tendency of overeating at meals time. You should have a snack 2 hours before your next scheduled meal. You have a lot of flexibility in what to choose for your snack.

Choose from:

Any raw vegetables (you can have them unlimited)
1 stick 2% fat mozzarella cheese
½ cup low-fat cottage cheese
½ cup fat-free humus
1-2 slices 2% fat cheese
½ cup part-skim ricotta cheese
½ cup berries
1 ounce almonds,
8 ounces low-fat low-sugar yogurt
½ cup grapefruit
1 orange
1 apple

Cottage Cheese Delight

1 small red onion, minced
1 tablespoon finely chopped, pimiento or parsley
1 carton (12 ounces) low-fat cottage cheese
Dash salt substitute

Combine cheese, onion, and salt .Beat well with electric mixer. Chill for one hour. Stir in pimiento or parsley. Serve with celery sticks.

Serves: 2

Guacamole

2 medium avocados, halved, seeded and pulp scooped out and cut up
1 tablespoon lemon juice
½ cup cherry tomatoes, chopped
½ green onion, finely chopped
1 tablespoon fresh parsley, chopped
½ cup tomatillo, chopped
1 garlic clove, minced
1 Anaheim pepper, seeded and finely chopped
¼ teaspoon salt substitute

Place avocado pulp in a medium bowl. Use a fork to mash the pulp, with the lemon juice, to make a chunky mixture. Stir in the rest of the ingredients. Cover and chill for 30 minutes before serving.
Serving suggestions: serve with raw vegetables.

Serves: 4

Romanian Style Eggplant Dip

1 medium eggplant, cut in half lengthwise
2 cloves garlic
½ white onion, finely chopped
2 tablespoon extra-virgin olive oil
1 teaspoon lemon juice
Salt substitute and ground black pepper to taste

Place eggplant cut side down and garlic gloves on a parchment-lined baking sheet. Roast the eggplant and garlic, in a preheated oven, at 375 degrees for 30 minutes, or until eggplant is soft to the touch. Remove from oven and cool. Peel eggplant and garlic. Place in a food processor; add onion, salt and black pepper. Puree until smooth. Add olive oil and pulse to incorporate the oil into eggplant puree.
Cool in refrigerator for 15 minutes before serving.
Serving suggestions: serve with raw vegetables.

Serves: 4

Cheese Bites

1 cup 2% fat white cheddar cheese, shredded
1 tablespoon fat-free cream cheese
1 tablespoon Smart Balance spread
½ cup whole wheat flour
¼ cup pitted black olives, chopped
½ cup egg substitute
2 tablespoons raw almonds, finely chopped
Dash ground black pepper

In a small mixing bowl, beat cheddar cheese, cream cheese, and spread, on low speed until blend. Add flour, black olives, black pepper and mix well. Beat in the egg substitute and almonds, until well combined. Spray a baking sheet with nonstick cooking spray and drop the mixture by teaspoonfuls. Bake at 400 degrees on preheated oven for 10 to 12 minutes or until golden brown.

Serves: 4

SIDE DISHES

Creamy Green Beans

1 package (9 ounces) frozen, cut green beans
½ cup water chestnuts, drained and sliced
½ cup green onion, finely chopped
1 cup fat-free sour cream
1 tablespoon Smart balance
1 clove garlic, minced
1 teaspoon salt substitute
Dash black pepper
1 tablespoon fresh dill, chopped

Cook beans according to package directions. Add chestnuts and heat through. Cook onion and garlic in 1 tablespoon Smart Balance, covered on low heat, until onion is translucent. Add remaining ingredients and heat through without boiling. Drain beans, and pour sauce over. Garnish with fresh dill.

Serves: 2

Broccoli Casserole

1 package (10 ounces) frozen chopped broccoli, cooked and drained
2 tablespoons Smart Balance
1 3-once fat-free cheese cream, softened
¼ cup crumbled blue cheese
1 cup fat-free milk
½ cup fat-free, sugar-free, whole wheat bread crumbs

In a sauce pan melt Smart Balance; blend in 2 tablespoon bread crumbs and cheese. Add milk and blue cheese, cook and stir until mixture boils. Stir in broccoli. Place in a 1-quart casserole, top with the remaining brad crumbs. Bake at 350 degrees for about 30 minutes.

Serves: 2

Company Cabbage

2 tablespoons olive oil
8 cups cabbage, finely shredded
1 clove garlic, minced
½ cup fat-free sour cream
2 tablespoons white vine vinegar
½ teaspoon salt substitute
Dash black pepper
1 tablespoon sesame seeds

Heat the oil in a large skillet. Add garlic, cabbage and ¼ cup water. Cover and steam over low heat for 15 minutes, stirring occasionally. Add salt, vinegar and pepper. Stir in sour cream. Heat all the way through without boiling. Sprinkle with sesame seeds.

Serves: 4

Cheese Cauliflower

1 medium head cauliflower
½ cup fat-free sour cream
2 teaspoons Dijon mustard
¾ cup 2% fat mild Cheddar cheese, shredded
1 teaspoon lemon juice
1 tablespoon chives
Dash black pepper

Remove leaves, and trim base from cauliflower. Wash, and boil in water for 15 minutes. ; drain. Place on un-greased shallow baking pan. Combine next ingredients except cheese, mix well and spread over cauliflower. Spread the cheese on top, and bake at 375 degrees until cheese is melted and bubbly.

Serves: 2

Ricotta Eggplant Rolls

1 large eggplant
2 cups part-skim ricotta cheese
1 cup egg substitute
2 tablespoons fresh parsley, chopped
Salt and ground black pepper to taste
1 cup bell peppers sauce
1 cup Michelle's tomato sauce (see recipe)

Cut stem and peel the eggplant. Cut lengthwise in ¼ inch slices. Spray a skillet with nonstick coking spray. Cook each eggplant slice until brown and tender on each side. Set aside on a plate. Mix well ricotta cheese, egg substitute, parsley, salt, and pepper. Spread one tablespoon of mixture evenly on each eggplant slice. Roll up and place seam side down on a sprayed baking dish. Mix bell pepper sauce and tomato sauce. Place one tablespoon on top of each eggplant roll.
If there is any sauce left, spread around in baking dish. Bake in oven at 400 degrees for 30 minutes. Serve warm.

Serves: 3

Oven Roasted Sweet Potatoes

1 medium sweet potato
1 small red onion, sliced
1 clove garlic, minced
Dash salt substitute
Dash black pepper

Pare, rinse sweet potato, and slice in ¼ inch rounds. Mix with next ingredients and place in a shallow baking pan sprayed with nonstick cooking spray. Cover with aluminum foil and bake at 400 degrees for 15 minutes stirring once. Uncover and bake for an additional 10 minutes or until tender.

Serves: 2

Oven Sweet Potatoes Fries

2 medium sweet potatoes
Dash salt substitute
Dash black pepper

Cut pared potatoes in half and then lengthwise in strips. Place potatoes strips on a Pam sprayed cookie sheet. Sprinkle with salt and pepper and spray once more with Pam.

Cover with aluminum foil and grill on low for 10 minutes. Uncover and grill for additional 5 minutes or until crisp. Flip over and brown other side. Serve at once.

Serves: 4

Scalloped Sweet Potatoes

2 medium sweet potatoes, pared and thinly sliced
2 tablespoon chopped scallions
2 clove garlic, minced
1 cup 2% fat mozzarella, shredded
1 cup fat-free milk
Dash salt substitute
Dash black pepper

Make a sauce mixing garlic, milk, cheese, salt, and pepper. Place half the potatoes in a Pam sprayed, 1-quart casserole; cover with half the onion and half the sauce. Repeat layers. Cover and bake at 350 degrees for about 45 minutes. Uncover and bake for an additional 15 minutes.

Serves: 4

Stuffed Sweet Potatoes

2 medium sweet potatoes
1 can (8 ounces) mushrooms, rinse and drained
1 small green pepper, finely chopped
1 scallion, finely chopped
1 clove garlic, minced
1 teaspoon Smart Balance
3 tablespoons fat-free milk

Bake potatoes in oven at 375 degrees. Cut slice from top of each. Scoop out the inside. Mash the pulp with Smart Balance, milk, garlic, salt, and black pepper to taste. Add onion, mushrooms and pepper. Fill shells with mixture. Return to oven and bake for additional 15 minutes at 375 degrees.

Serves: 4

Mashed Sweet Potatoes

2 large sweet potatoes
1 cup fat-free milk
1 tablespoon fat-free sour cream
1 clove garlic, minced
2 tablespoon fresh parsley chopped
Dash salt substitute
Dash black pepper

Boil sweet potatoes until fork-tender. Peel while still hot and mash. Beat until fluffy, gradually adding hot milk. Beat in garlic, salt, pepper, and sour cream. Sprinkle with fresh parsley before serving.

Serves: 4

Double Baked Sweet Potatoes

2 medium sweet potatoes
½ cup 2% fat cedar cheese, shredded
½ cup part-skim mozzarella cheese, shredded
¼ cup green onion, finely chopped
¼ cup grape tomatoes, finely chopped
¼ teaspoon black pepper
1 clove garlic, minced
¼ teaspoon paprika
2 tablespoon fresh cilantro, chopped

Preheat oven at 400 degrees. Wash potatoes and pierce with fork in several places. Bake potatoes for 35 minutes or until fork-tender. Remove from oven and cool.

Reduce oven temperature to 325 degrees. Slice potatoes in half lengthwise. Scoop out most of the potato pulp, forming four shells. Mash potato pulp; add cedar cheese, mozzarella cheese, onion, garlic, paprika and black pepper. Blend until smooth; add tomatoes and cilantro; mix until well blended. Fill shells with equal amounts of potato mixture. Wrap skin in foil leaving tops open. Place on baking sheet and bake for 20 minutes. Serve hot.

Serves: 4

Onion Sweet Potatoes

2 large sweet potatoes
1 tablespoon fresh lemon juice
1 tablespoon olive oil
1 medium red onion
1 tablespoon fresh parsley, chopped
1 teaspoon salt substitute

Peel sweet potatoes, wash and cut into 1 inch strips, than cut across into cubes. Boil potatoes in salted water, until tender; when almost done add lemon juice; drain and place potatoes on a serving plate. Peel, wash and chop the onion. Add oil to a skillet and sauté onion until golden. Put onion over potatoes. Sprinkle with fresh parsley.

Serves: 4

Sweet Potatoes Sauté

2 large sweet potatoes
1 tablespoon olive oil
½ teaspoon salt substitute
½ teaspoon ground black pepper
¼ teaspoon nutmeg
2 tablespoon fresh parsley, chopped

Boil potatoes in salted water until fork tender. Drain and cool. Peel skin off, and shred the potatoes. Put olive oil in a large skillet; place over medium heat. Add potatoes to skillet. Sprinkle with salt, black pepper, nutmeg, and sauté until golden. Sprinkle with fresh parsley.

Serves: 4

Sauerkraut Sweet Potatoes

1 can (16 ounces) Sauerkraut
2 sweet potatoes
2 medium ripe tomatoes, peeled and chopped
½ teaspoon salt substitute
½ teaspoon ground black pepper
1 teaspoon dry oregano
2 tablespoons olive oil

Wash sauerkraut thoroughly; drain. Boil potatoes in skin until fork tender. Cool, peel and cut potatoes in thin slices. In pan heat oil, add sauerkraut and cook uncovered over medium heat until golden. Add 2 cups cold water, and cook covered, stirring occasionally, for 30 minutes. Uncover and cook over low heat until all water evaporates. Add tomatoes and potatoes to pan. Add salt, pepper and oregano. Stir and cook for additional 5 minutes.

Serves: 4

Brussels sprouts Sauté

1½ pond Brussels sprouts
1 medium white onion, chopped
2 tablespoons olive oil
2 cups red dry wine
1 tablespoon fresh chives
½ teaspoon salt substitute
½ teaspoon ground black pepper

Remove any discolored leaves from the Brussels sprouts, and cut off stem ends. Wash sprouts and cut in half. Heat oil in shallow pan; add onion and cook until translucent. Add sprouts and sauté for 15 minutes. Add salt, pepper, and wine; cover and cook over low heat until sprouts are fork tender. Uncover and cook until sauce reduces. Sprinkle with chives before serving.

Serves: 2

Grandma's Cabbage

1 large cabbage
4 medium white onions, chopped
1 teaspoon caraway
1 cup dry white wine
1 tablespoon soy flour
2 tablespoons olive oil
¼ teaspoon ground black pepper
1 teaspoon salt substitute
1 tablespoon low-fat sour cream

Wash cabbage, shred and boil in salted water for 15 minutes; drain. In large pan heat oil, add onion, and cook until translucent. Add cabbage, caraway, salt, pepper and wine. Cook covered over low heat, until cabbage is tender. Mix soy flour, sour cream and 1 tablespoon cold water; pour over cabbage and stir. Cover and cook in oven at 375 degrees for 15 to 20 minutes.

Serves: 4

Fried Eggplant

2 medium eggplants
4 medium ripe tomatoes, peeled and chopped
1 green bell pepper, chopped
1 tablespoon fresh parsley, chopped
1 tablespoon olive oil
3 garlic cloves, minced
1 teaspoon salt substitute
¼ teaspoon ground black pepper

Cut off stem ends from eggplant. Wash and cut the eggplant in ½ inch slices. Salt and let it stand for 1 hour. Press between 2 paper towels to drain. Spray a skillet with nonstick cooking spray and fry eggplant slices on both sides until golden. Place eggplant slices in a baking pan. In a skillet put tomatoes, bell pepper, garlic, salt and black pepper; sauté for 5 minutes. Put mixture over eggplant slices. Cook over low heat for 10 minutes. Sprinkle on top with fresh parsley before serving.

Serves: 4

Zucchini Patties

2 medium zucchini
½ cup white onion, grated
1 clove garlic, minced
¼ cup egg substitute
1 teaspoon salt substitute
¼ teaspoon black pepper
1 tablespoon fresh parsley, chopped

Peel zucchini and grate. Squeeze out all liquid. In a bowl mix well all ingredients. Shape into round patties. Spray a skillet with nonstick cooking spray and place over medium heat. Add patties to the skillet, and fry for 5 to 7 minutes on each side, turning once.

Serves: 2

Cauliflower Casserole

1 large cauliflower
1 cup fat-free sour cream
1 cup egg substitute
1 tablespoon Smart Balance spread
1 cup fat-free Feta cheese, crumbled
1 tablespoon light rye bread crumbs
1 teaspoon salt substitute
Dash ground black pepper

Cook cauliflower flowerets in boiling salted water for 10 minutes. Drain. Mix well egg substitute with sour cream, salt, and ground black pepper. Coat a baking pan with Smart Balance spread and bread crumbs. Place cauliflower flowerets in the pan; pour the sauce over, and sprinkle the cheese on top. Bake in the oven at 350 degrees for 20 minutes or until the top is golden, and sauce bubbles at sides.

Serves: 3

Brussels sprouts Casserole

2 pounds Brussels sprouts
1 tablespoon Smart Balance spread
1 cup part-skim mozzarella cheese, shredded
1 tablespoon fat-free sour cream
Salt and black pepper to taste

Boil sprouts in salted water until tender; drain. Coat a baking pan with Smart Balance spread. Put half of cheese at the bottom of the pan. Add sprouts, and the other half of cheese. Spread sour cream on top. Bake in oven at 350 degrees for 10 minutes until golden brown.

Serves: 4

Red Cabbage Sauté

1 medium red cabbage
1 red onion, chopped
1 cup red dry wine
1 cup water
1 teaspoon salt substitute
½ teaspoon whole black pepper
1 tablespoon Smart Balance spread

Shred the cabbage. Sauté onion in Smart Balance spread until onion is translucent. Add cabbage, salt, pepper and wine. Cook over low heat for one hour.

Serves: 3

Sauerkraut and Olives Delight

1 can (16ounces) sauerkraut
1 tablespoon olive oil
1can (6ounces) black olives
1 teaspoon paprika
1 teaspoon savory
1 medium white onion, finely chopped

Rinse and drain sauerkraut. In a large skillet, sauté onion in olive oil, until onion is translucent. Add sauerkraut, paprika, savory, and 1 cup cold water. Cover and cook for 30 minutes over low heat stirring occasionally. Add black olives and cook for additional 10 minutes.

Serves: 2

Cabbage Patties

1 medium cabbage, finely shredded
1 tablespoon Smart Balance spread
2 tablespoons fat-free sour cream
2 tablespoons light rye bread crumbs
1 teaspoon salt substitute
½ teaspoon ground black pepper
1 cup egg substitute

Boil cabbage in salted water for 10 minutes; drain. Sauté cabbage in Smart Balance spread for 5 minutes stirring constantly; cool. Mix well cabbage, egg substitute, sour cream, salt, black pepper and bread crumbs. In a sauce pan bring water to a boil. Place one full tablespoon, of cabbage mixture, at the time in the boiling water. Boil for 3 minutes each. Serve hot with fat-free sour cream.

Serves: 3

Spinach Casserole

2 pounds fresh spinach
3 tablespoons part-skim mozzarella cheese, shredded
1 tablespoon Smart Balance spread
½ tablespoon barley flour
Dash salt substitute
Dash ground black pepper
1 cup fat-free vegetable broth

Blanch spinach in salted water. Drain and chop finely. In a large pan put ½ tablespoon Smart Balance, flour and spinach; mix well. Add vegetable broth and cook over low heat for 15 minutes stirring frequently. Put aside. Coat a baking pan with ½ tablespoon Smart Balance. Add salt, black pepper and 2 tablespoons mozzarella cheese to spinach; mix well. Put spinach in baking pan, sprinkle 1 tablespoon mozzarella cheese on top and bake in oven at 375 degrees for 15 minutes or until top is golden brown.

Serves: 2

Creamy Zucchini

6 medium zucchini
1 tablespoon Smart Balance spread
1 cup fat-free sour cream
1 teaspoon whole grain flour
1 cup part-skim mozzarella cheese, shredded
Dash salt
Dash ground black pepper

Peel zucchini and cut in half lengthwise. Blanch in salted water and drain. Heat a skillet; add Smart Balance spread and zucchini; cover and sauté for 5 minutes. Mix flour, salt, black pepper and sour cream. Put zucchini in a baking pan, pour over sour cream mixture, and sprinkle on top mozzarella cheese. Bake in oven at 375 degrees for 20 minutes.

Serves: 3

Zucchini and Tomatoes Casserole

3 medium zucchini
3 medium tomatoes, thin sliced
6 oz. Farmers Cheese, thin sliced
1 tablespoon Smart Balance
Dash salt
Dash ground black pepper
1 cup part-skim mozzarella cheese, shredded

Peel zucchini and slice into 1/8 inch rounds. Coat a skillet with non stick cooking spray and fry zucchini rounds on each side until golden. Set aside. Coat a baking pan with Smart Balance spread. Put one layer of zucchini, one layer of tomatoes, and one layer of cheese. Repeat, the layers until all vegetables are gone. Sprinkle mozzarella cheese on top and bake in oven at 350 degrees for 30 minutes.

Serves: 2

Cheese Stuffed Zucchini

6 medium zucchini
1 tablespoon Smart Balance spread
2 tablespoons fat-free Feta cheese, crumbled
1 tablespoon whole grain bread crumbs
2 tablespoons fat-free sour cream
Dash salt substitute
Dash ground black pepper
1 tablespoon fresh parsley, chopped
1 cup reduction tomato sauce

Peel zucchini and cut in half cross wise; scoop out pulp leaving ¼ inch wall. Chop pulp and sauté in Smart Balance for 10 minutes, over low heat. Set aside. Mix well pulp, Feta cheese, salt, black pepper, parsley and bread crumbs. Fill zucchini halves with mixture. Place halves in a baking pan. Mix well tomato sauce and sour cream. Pour sauce over zucchini and bake at 350 degrees for 30 minutes or until zucchini are tender. Do not over cook.

Serves: 6

Green Beans in Tomato Sauce

2 pounds green beans
1 medium white onion, chopped
1 tablespoon olive oil
1 tablespoon fresh parsley, chopped
½ teaspoon dried oregano
2 cups reduction tomato sauce

Boil green beans for 10 minutes; drain. In a skillet, sauté the onion in olive oil, until tender. In a baking pan put green beans, onion, parsley, oregano, and tomato sauce. Mix well and cook in oven for 30 minutes at 375 degrees.

Serves: 4

Mashed Lentils

1 pound lentils
2 white onions, finely chopped
1 tablespoon olive oil
1 teaspoon salt substitute
½ teaspoon ground black pepper
2 cups fat-free vegetable broth
1 clove garlic, minced
1 teaspoon fresh cilantro, chopped

Keep lentils for 1 hour in warm water; rinse thoroughly. Boil lentils in vegetable broth on low heat until soft (add water if needed). Drain and mashed. Add salt substitute, black pepper and cilantro; mix well. Meanwhile heat a skillet, add olive oil, garlic and onion; cook over low heat until onion is golden brown. Spread cooked onion on top.

Serves: 2

Mushrooms Stuffed Tomatoes

6 big tomatoes
1 pound fresh mushrooms
2 medium red onions, finely chopped
1 tablespoon extra virgin olive oil
1 teaspoon red Bell pepper paste
1 garlic clove, minced
1 tablespoon whole grain bread crumbs
1 teaspoon salt substitute
½ teaspoon ground black pepper
1 tablespoon fresh parsley, chopped
1 cup cold water
½ cup part-skim mozzarella cheese, shredded
1 cup tomato juice

Cut tomatoes in half lengthwise; scoop out some of the pulp and seeds. Peel skin off mushrooms and chop. Coat a skillet with nonstick cooking spray; add onion and cook on low heat until translucent. Add mushrooms and cook until mushrooms are tender. Add 1 teaspoon red Bell pepper paste, minced garlic, salt, black pepper, fresh parsley, whole grain bread crumbs and water. Cook over low heat until thickens. Fill tomato halves with mixture. Place tomato halves in baking pan. Sprinkle mozzarella cheese on top of each tomato half. Mix olive oil and tomato juice and add it to pan. Bake in oven at 350 degrees for 30 minutes or until tomatoes are tender; do not overcook.

Serves: 6

Mushrooms in Sauce Piquant

1 pound Shiitake mushrooms
3 small white onions, chopped
2 tablespoons olive oil
½ cup dry red wine
½ teaspoon ground black pepper
1 tablespoon fresh dill weed, chopped
1 tablespoon fresh lemon juice
½ teaspoon salt substitute
½ chili, chopped

Wash mushrooms and slice. Put olive oil in a sauce pan and place over low heat. Add onion and sauté until onion is golden. Add mushrooms and cook over low heat for 15 to 20 minutes. Add wine, lemon juice, salt, chili, black pepper and dill weed. Bring to a boil and boil for 3 minutes.
Serving suggestion: serve cold, garnish with tomato slices.

Serves: 2

Easy Asparagus

1 pound asparagus, washed and trimmed
1 tablespoon olive oil
4 garlic cloves, minced
Salt and ground black pepper to taste
1 tablespoon red wine vinegar

Combine oil, vinegar, salt, black pepper and garlic in a bowl. Add asparagus and toss to coat. Cover and refrigerate for 30 minutes. Heat a flat grill for searing. Put asparagus on grill and sear for about 5 minutes. Turn and sear for additional 5 minutes or until asparagus is fork tender.
Serve warm, with grilled fish.

Serves: 2

Easy Broccoli

1 pound broccoli flowerets
1 tablespoon extra-virgin olive oil
1 tablespoon lemon juice
3 cloves garlic, minced
1 tablespoon fresh parsley
Salt substitute and black pepper to taste

Boil broccoli flowerets in salted water for 5 minutes; drain. Put rest of the ingredients in a food processor, and mix well. Pour sauce over broccoli and serve.

Serves: 2

Refreshing Salsa

2 medium tomatoes cut in half
6 tomatillos
1 medium red onion, finely chopped
1 fresh Serrano pepper, seeded and finely chopped
1 clove garlic, minced
2 tablespoons fresh parsley, chopped

Place tomatoes cut sides down, on broiler pan. Broil 4 inches from heat for 10 minutes or until tomato skins start to blacken. Remove from broiler pan and cool. Remove skin from tomatoes and chop. Remove husks from fresh tomatillos and rinse. Chop finely. In a bowl, stir together chopped tomatillos, chopped grilled tomatoes, onion, parsley, Serrano pepper and salt substitute to taste. Cover and chill for 3 hours before serving.
Serving suggestion: Serve over grille fish or grilled chicken breast.

Serves: 4

Green Beans Sauté

2 pounds fresh green bean
1 medium white onion, finely chopped
2 tablespoons olive oil
1 tablespoon fresh parsley, chopped
1 tablespoon fresh dill weed, chopped
1 teaspoon Dijon mustard
2 tablespoons lemon juice
1 teaspoon salt substitute
¼ teaspoon ground black pepper

Boil green beans in salted water until tender. Drain and place in a salad bowl. Mix well all the ingredients. Pour over green beans and toss to coat. Cover and refrigerate for 2 hours before serving.

Serves: 3

Eggplant Portuguese

4 medium eggplants
6 oz. Farmers cheese, thin sliced
1 tablespoon olive oil
2 medium white onions, chopped
1 pound fresh tomatoes, sliced
2 garlic cloves, minced
1 teaspoon allspice
2 bay leaves
1 teaspoon salt substitute
½ teaspoon ground black pepper
1 tablespoon fresh parsley, chopped
1 cup part-skim mozzarella cheese, shredded

Slice eggplant in ¼ inch rounds and blanch in salted water; drain and press for 20 minutes. Heat a large skillet; add olive oil and onion; cook onion over low heat until translucent. Add tomatoes, garlic, allspice, bay leaves, salt and black pepper, to the pan. Cover and boil over low heat for 30 minutes until sauce is thickened; strain. Pat dry eggplant rounds with paper towel. Coat a skillet with nonstick cooking spray, place over medium heat, and fry each eggplant round on each side until golden brown. Place in a casserole dish a layer of sauce, a layer of cheese, a layer of eggplant; repeat until you use all eggplant rounds. Last layer should be sauce. Sprinkle mozzarella cheese on top. Garnish with parsley. Bake in oven at 375 degrees for 25 minutes until top is lightly browned and bubbly.

Serves: 4

Vegetables Hotchpotch

1 sweet potato
3 small zucchini
1 parsnip, peeled and sliced
2 parsley roots, peeled and sliced
1 small eggplant, sliced
4 ripe tomatoes, sliced
3 green bell peppers, sliced

1 small cabbage, finely sliced
4 medium red onions, chopped
1 pound green beans
3 garlic cloves, minced
1 small celery root, peeled and sliced
2 tablespoons olive oil
½ teaspoon whole black peppercorns
1 teaspoon salt substitute
1 tablespoon fresh cilantro, chopped

Peel zucchini and sweet potato. Wash and cube. In a large sauce pan add oil, and place over low heat; add onion, parsnip, parsley roots, bell peppers and cabbage. Sauté for 10 minutes stirring occasionally. Add zucchini and sweet potato to the pan. Blanch green beans in salted water. Drain and add to the sauce pan. Add rest of vegetables: eggplant, and garlic. Add black peppercorns and salt. Cook over low heat for 40 minutes stirring occasionally. Add tomato slices and cook for additional 10 minutes. Sprinkle cilantro on top before serving.

Serves: 4

Mushrooms Goulash

2 pounds fresh mushrooms
2 tablespoons olive oil
2 medium white onions, chopped
1 tablespoon paprika
1 teaspoon salt substitute

Peel skin off mushrooms, wash and cut in half. Heat oil in a large skillet; add onion and cook until translucent. Add mushrooms and cook for 10 minutes; add paprika salt and water just enough to cover mushrooms. Cook uncovered for 15 minutes.

Serves: 2

Cauliflower Goulash

1 medium cauliflower
2 tablespoon olive oil
1 large red onion, finely chopped
1 teaspoon paprika
1 teaspoon salt substitute
½ teaspoon ground black pepper
1 teaspoon white wine vinegar

Separate cauliflower into flowerets. Put flowerets in water with vinegar, and let it stand for 10 minutes; drain. In large pan cook the onion, until is translucent. Add paprika, salt, black pepper, and 1 cup cold water. Add cauliflower flowerets and cook covered over low heat until cauliflower is fork tender.

Serves: 2

Andra's Cauliflower Delight

1 medium cauliflower, separated in flowerets and steamed
1 medium white onion, chopped
1 ½ cup low-fat sour cream
3 garlic cloves, minced
½ cup part-skim mozzarella cheese, shredded
¼ teaspoon ground black pepper

Coat a skillet with nonstick cooking spray. Place over medium heat. Add onion and garlic to the skillet and cook until golden brown. Remove from heat. In a bowl mix sour cream, cheese and black pepper. Add cooked onion and garlic to the bowl. Add steamed cauliflower flowerets. Toss well to coat. Serve immediately.

Serves: 2

Eggplant and Zucchini Parmigiana

1 medium eggplant
2 medium zucchini
2 cups Michelle's tomato sauce (see recipe)
½ teaspoon oregano
1 tablespoon fresh parsley, chopped
1 8-oz. Ricotta cheese (part-skim)
½ cup grated Parmesan
Salt and ground black pepper to taste

Wash eggplant and cut into ½ inch thick slices. Coat a skillet with nonstick cooking spray and place over medium heat. Add eggplant slices to the skillet and fry until brown and tender flipping once. Do the same with zucchini. Mix tomato sauce with oregano and parsley. Coat a 2 quart casserole with nonstick cooking spray. Place eggplant and zucchini slices in layers, alternating with sauce, seasonings and ricotta cheese. Sprinkle on top with Parmesan cheese. Bake at 375 degrees for 30 to 40 minutes.

Serves: 2

Garlic Lima Beans

2 cans (5.5 ounces), lima beans
2 tablespoons olive oil
2 garlic cloves, minced
1 teaspoon Dijon mustard
1 tablespoon white wine vinegar
1 tablespoon fresh parsley, chopped
1 teaspoon salt substitute
¼ teaspoon ground black pepper

Wash and drain lima beans. Heat the olive oil in large skillet. Add garlic and Lima beans; cover and sauté for 10 minutes over low heat. Pull away from heat. Mix well vinegar, mustard, salt and pepper. Pour sauce over lima beans end toss to coat. Sprinkle with fresh parsley.

Serves: 2

Mushrooms Delight

2 pounds Portobello mushrooms
2 tablespoons Smart Balance spread
¼ teaspoon ground black pepper
1 tablespoon dill weed, chopped
1 teaspoon salt substitute
3 tablespoons dry white wine
¼ teaspoon nutmeg

Peel mushrooms, wash and chop. In a pan put spread, mushrooms, and 1 cup cold water; cover and cook for 20 minutes over low heat. Add salt, wine and half tablespoon of dill weed. Boil for additional 10 minutes. Pull away from heat. Add nutmeg, black pepper and the other half tablespoon of dill weed.

Serves: 2

Tomato Beets

3 medium beets
3 medium white onions, chopped
2 parsley roots
3 medium ripe tomatoes, peeled and chopped
2 tablespoons olive oil
1 teaspoon salt substitute
½ teaspoon ground black pepper
1 tablespoon fresh parsley, chopped

Peel beets and parsley roots; wash and chop. Heat oil in a large skillet; add onion and cook over low heat until translucent. Add beets and parsley to the skillet, and cook covered, until vegetables are fork tender. Add tomatoes, salt and pepper and cook for additional 15 minutes. Sprinkle with fresh parsley before serving.

Serves: 4

Row Beet Salad

2 medium beets
1 medium horseradish root
1 teaspoon red wine vinegar
1 teaspoon Smart Balance spread
1 teaspoon salt substitute
¼ teaspoon ground black pepper
1 teaspoon ground caraway

Peel, wash and shred beets. Peel horseradish root and shred finely. Mix beets and horseradish. In a sauce pan, melt Smart Balance spread; add salt, pepper, caraway and vinegar; mix well; pour sauce over beets and toss well to coat.

Serves: 3

Oven Roasted Vegetables

1 medium red onion, sliced
4 garlic cloves, minced
1 red bell pepper, sliced
1 green bell pepper, sliced
1 zucchini, sliced
1 yellow squash, sliced
½ teaspoon salt substitute
½ teaspoon fresh ground black pepper
¼ teaspoon dry oregano
1 tablespoon extra-virgin, cold press olive oil

Preheat oven to 400 degrees. Season vegetables and toss to coat evenly. Spray a roasting pan with nonstick cooking spray. Add vegetables to the pan and roast for 20 minutes or until vegetables are fork tender.
Serving suggestion: with grilled tuna steak or grilled salmon and sauce piquant.

Serves: 2

Vegetables Sauté

1 medium zucchini cut in ½ inch cubes
1 medium yellow squash cut in ½ inch cubes
1 small red onion chopped
1 cup grape tomatoes, chopped
1 teaspoon olive oil
4 garlic cloves, minced
2 tablespoons fresh parsley, chopped
¼ teaspoon dried oregano
2 tablespoons dried cranberry
1 tablespoon caper
¼ teaspoon nutmeg
2 tablespoons pitted black olives, sliced
Salt and black pepper to taste

Heat the oil, in a large skillet over medium heat. Add onion and garlic; cook for 2 minutes. Add zucchini and yellow squash, and cook for additional 2 minutes. Add remaining ingredients except black olive and parsley. Stir, cover, and simmer on low heat for 15 minutes. Add black olives and parsley. Stir, and cook uncovered for 5 minutes.

Serves: 2

Celery in Tomato Sauce

2 celery roots
1 medium white onion, chopped
1 cup reduction tomato sauce
1 garlic clove minced
1 tablespoon fresh parsley, chopped

Peel celery roots; wash thoroughly and slice in ¼ inch rounds. Spray a skillet with nonstick cooking spray and place over low heat; add celery rounds to skillet and cook on each side until golden; set aside. Coat a skillet with nonstick cooking spray, and sauté the onion, over low heat, until tender. Add garlic, tomato sauce and ½ cup cold water and bring to a boil. Place celery rounds in a baking dish; pour sauce over, and cook in the oven at 350 degrees for 30 minutes. Garnish with parsley before serving.

Serves: 2

Celery and Mushrooms Delight

3 medium celery roots
2 medium white onions, chopped
14 oz. fresh mushrooms, peeled, washed and chopped
½ cup dry white wine
1 teaspoon salt substitute
Dash ground black pepper
2 bay leaves
1 tablespoon fresh parsley, chopped
1 tablespoon Smart Balance spread

Peel, wash and slice celery roots in ¼ inch rounds. Boil celery rounds in salted water until tender; drain. Sauté onion in 1 tablespoon spread until onion is tender; add wine, ½ cup cold water, salt, pepper and bay leaves. Boil over low heat for 20 minutes; set aside and discard bay leaves. Spray a skillet with nonstick cooking spray; place over medium heat and sauté mushrooms until tender.

In a sauce pan put celery rounds, mushrooms and pour sauce over. Boil for 20 minutes over low heat. Garnish with parsley before serving.

Serves: 3

Garlic Stuffed Onion

6 medium white onions
2 garlic bulbs
1 tablespoon olive oil
1 teaspoon salt substitute
¼ teaspoon ground black pepper
1 teaspoon light rye bread crumbs

Blanch onions and garlic bulbs; drain. Cut ¼ inch from top of each onion and carefully scoop out pulp leaving ¼ inch wall.

Peel skin of garlic and press. Mix well pressed garlic, chopped onion pulp, salt, black pepper and ½ tablespoon olive oil. Fill onions with mixture; sprinkle on top with bread crumbs. Put the other half tablespoon of olive oil in a baking dish; add filled onions and bake in oven at 375 degrees until golden.

Serving suggestions: steak, grilled chicken breast, oven roasted sweet potatoes.

Serves: 6

Roasted Peppers Salad I

3 large red bell peppers
3 large yellow bell peppers
2 cloves garlic, finely sliced
1 teaspoon salt substitute
2 tablespoons red wine vinegar
2 tablespoons cold water

Coat a broiler pan with nonstick cooking spray. Place peppers on pan and broil 5 inch from top turning occasionally, until skin is evenly browned and blistered. Place peppers in a plastic bag and close tightly; let stand for about 20 minutes, and then remove skin, stems and seeds. Place peppers in a glass, serving bowl. Mix well garlic, salt, vinegar and water; pour over peppers. Cover and refrigerate for at least 2 hours before serving.

Serves: 6

Cucumbers Salad

1 medium cucumber, skinless, seedless
½ cup fat-free sour cream
1 tablespoon white wine vinegar
1 tablespoon snipped chives
1 clove garlic, minced
1 teaspoon dill weed
Dash black pepper
Dash salt substitute

Slice cucumber in thin slices; sprinkle with salt and let it stand for 15 minutes; drain.

Mix next ingredients and pour over cucumbers. Chill before serving for 30 minutes.

Serves: 2

Roasted Peppers Salad II

6 yellow bell peppers
4 medium tomatoes
1 tablespoon fresh dill weed, chopped
2 tablespoons cold water
1 tablespoon olive oil
1 tablespoon white wine vinegar
1 teaspoon salt substitute

Place bell peppers on rack in broiler pan. Broil with tops about 5 inches from heat, turning occasionally until skin is blistered and evenly browned. Place peppers in a plastic bag and let stand for 20 minutes. Remove skin, steams and seeds from peppers. Place in a salad bowl. Cut tomatoes in thin round slices; place over bell peppers. Sprinkle on top dill weed. Mix well olive oil, vinegar, water and salt. Pour sauce over peppers and tomatoes.

Serves: 6

Tomato Salad I

3 green bell peppers
3 medium tomatoes
1 cucumber
1 tablespoon olive oil
2 teaspoon fresh dill weed, chopped
1 tablespoon red wine vinegar
½ teaspoon salt substitute

Remove steams and seeds from bell peppers, wash and cut in thin slices. Cut tomatoes in thin slices. Peel cucumber, cut in half lengthwise, remove seeds and cut in thin slices. Place tomatoes, peppers, and cucumbers in a salad bowl. Add olive oil, dill weed, vinegar, and salt. Toss to coat and serve.

Serves: 3

Tomato Salad II

3 medium cucumbers
3 medium tomatoes
1 tablespoon olive oil
2 garlic cloves, minced
1 tablespoon white wine vinegar
1 tablespoon cold water
1 teaspoon fresh dill weed, chopped
1 teaspoon salt substitute
Dash ground black pepper

Peel cucumbers and cut in half lengthwise; remove seeds and cut in ¼ inch slices. Cut tomatoes in thin slices. Place tomatoes and cucumbers in a salad bowl. Mix well garlic, vinegar, olive oil, dill weed, salt, black pepper and water. Pour sauce over tomatoes and cucumbers, and toss to coat.

Serves: 4

Mushroom Salad

15 big mushrooms
1 tablespoon olive oil
1 teaspoon white wine vinegar
1 tablespoon red wine vinegar
¼ teaspoon ground black pepper
1 teaspoon salt substitute
1 teaspoon fresh parsley, chopped

Wash mushrooms, and boil in salted water with 1 teaspoon white vinegar for 15 minutes. Drain; save the water and let it cool. Slice mushrooms and place in a salad bowl. Mix well water, salt, black pepper, red vinegar and parsley. Pour sauce over mushrooms. Toss and chill for half hour before serving.

Serves: 4

Peppers and Tomato Relish

4 green bell peppers
3 medium red onions, sliced
3 medium ripe tomatoes, peeled and chopped
2 tablespoons olive oil
1 tablespoon fresh parsley, chopped
1 teaspoon salt substitute
½ teaspoon ground black pepper
1 red pepper, chopped

Remove stems and seeds from bell peppers. Wash and slice. Add oil to a skillet; place over low heat. Add onion and cook until tender. Add bell peppers, tomatoes, red pepper, salt and black pepper. Boil for 20 minutes over low heat or until vegetables are tender, stirring occasionally. Sprinkle with fresh parsley.
Serving suggestions: grilled steak, grilled or boiled chicken breast, and grilled fish.

Michelle's Tomato Sauce

10 large tomatoes
4 celery stalks
8 garlic cloves
2 tablespoons fresh parsley, chopped
4 basil leaves
1 cup fat-free, low-sodium vegetable broth.

Cut tomatoes in fourths. Cut celery in fourths. Put all the ingredients, less basil leaves, in a blender (if you don't have a food processor) and pure. Put tomato sauce in a sauce pan; add basil leaves and boil over low heat for 2 hours. Cool and store in jars. I found that jelly jars are perfect to store this sauce.
Serving suggestion: great for Moussaka, over grilled eggplant, meat balls, and oven roasted sweet potatoes.

Tomato Sauce

2 cups, low-sugar, tomato juice
1 tablespoon tomato paste
½ dry white wine
1 tablespoon olive oil
1 teaspoon dry savory
1 teaspoon salt substitute

Mix tomato juice and tomato paste together, and boil for ten minutes, over low heat. Add vine, salt, and savory. Boil for another five minutes, over low heat.
Serving suggestion: with grilled fish, and steamed green beans, grilled steak.

Tarragon Sauce

1 cup light mayonnaise
1 tablespoon fresh tarragon, chopped
2 teaspoon fresh parsley, chopped
2 small white onions, finely chopped
1 small pickle
¼ teaspoon ground black pepper

Chop pickle finely and dry it in a paper towel. Mix well all the ingredients. Cool for ½ hour before serving.
Serving suggestion: with baked or grilled fish.

Garlic Sauce I

1 large garlic bulb
1 teaspoon salt substitute
1 tablespoon olive oil
1 tablespoon red wine vinegar
2 tablespoons cold water

Peel the skin off the garlic and minced. Put garlic in a small bowl. Add salt and oil a little bit at the time while mixing constantly until it looks like a mayonnaise. Stir in vinegar and water.
Serving suggestion: with oven sweet potatoes fries, grilled fish, boiled chicken breast, and steamed vegetables.

Garlic Sauce II

1 garlic bulb, peeled and minced
1 teaspoon salt substitute
1 cup fat-free, low-sodium, vegetable broth

Mix well all ingredients.
Serving suggestion: grilled fish, boiled meat, and grilled vegetables.

Sauce Piquant

5 green bell peppers
5 red bell peppers
6 medium tomatoes
3 medium white onions
3 tablespoon olive oil
1 tablespoon red wine vinegar
5 garlic cloves
1 teaspoon salt substitute
1 red chili pepper
2 tablespoon cold water
1 teaspoon ground black pepper

Peel, wash, and chop onion. In a large skillet add olive oil, onion, and cook over low heat until onion is tender. Add bell peppers finely sliced, and chili pepper chopped to the pan. Cover and simmer for 5 minutes. Add tomatoes, peeled and chopped, salt, black pepper, minced garlic, vinegar, and water; mix well. Cook over low heat for 25 minutes, stirring frequently.
Serving suggestion: with grilled or baked chicken breast, beef steak, and steamed vegetables.

Sauce Vinaigrette

2 tablespoons olive oil
4 tablespoons red wine vinegar
2 garlic cloves, minced
½ teaspoon Dijon mustard
½ teaspoon salt substitute

In a small bowl mix well all ingredients. This is a very good salad dressing. You can make more at the time, and keep it refrigerated.

Red Bell Pepper Sauce

9 large bell peppers
6 garlic cloves, minced
1 teaspoon black peppercorn
3 dry bay leaves

Remove stem and seeds from peppers, and cut the peppers in forth. Put peppers and garlic in a food processor and puree. Pour the obtained sauce in a large sauce pan; place over low heat and boil for 30 minutes stirring frequently. Add black pepper and bay leaves. Continue to boil for another 30 minutes. Discard bay leaves.
Let it cool and pour sauce in jelly jars. Refrigerate until using.
Serving suggestions: with grilled fish and grilled chicken breast.

Delicious Salad Dressing

¼ cup egg substitute, well beaten
½ teaspoon salt substitute
¼ teaspoon ground black pepper
½ teaspoon Dijon mustard
¼ cup white wine vinegar
½ cup 2% fat milk
1 teaspoon Splenda sugar substitute

Mix all ingredients in a sauce pan. Place over low heat and simmer for 10 minutes stirring constantly. Remove form heat and cool. Refrigerate until using.

Blue Cheese Salad Dressing

1 cup low-fat plain yogurt
½ cup low-fat sour cream
1 cup blue cheese, crumbled
1 tablespoon fresh parsley, chopped
2 cloves garlic, chopped
¼ teaspoon ground black pepper
Salt substitute to taste

Put all ingredients in a blender. Blend until smooth. Refrigerate for 20 minutes before using.

DESERTS

Cottage Cheese Soufflé

1 carton (16 ounces) fat-free cottage cheese
1 cup egg substitute
1½ tablespoons Splenda sugar substitute
3 tablespoon fat-free sour cream
½ cup whole wheat flour
Pinch salt
1 teaspoon cinnamon
2 egg whites, stiffly beaten
1 tablespoon Smart Balance spread

Preheat oven at 350 degrees. Melt Smart Balance spread in a 1-quart pan until it sizzles. Remove from heat and add cheese, sour cream, and salt. Mix well. Blend in the flour. Incorporate egg substitute and fold in the egg whites. Pour into individual soufflé dishes. Sprinkle with cinnamon and bake for one hour.

Serves: 2

Strawberries Salad

½ pound fresh strawberries
2 teaspoon Splenda sugar substitute
1 tablespoon walnuts, chopped
1 teaspoon fresh lemon juice
1 apple, boiled and sliced

Wash the strawberries, and remove the stems. Drain and cut in half. Place the strawberries in a salad bowl. Add apple slices, lemon juice, sugar substitute and nuts, to the bowl. Toss to coat evenly. Place the strawberries salad into serving cups. Refrigerate for ½ hour before serving.

Serves: 2

Fruit Salad

10 strawberries, cubed
½ apple, cubed
2 tablespoons cantaloupe, cubed
1 tablespoon blueberries
1 tablespoon fresh lemon juice
1 tablespoon Splenda sugar substitute
1 teaspoon rum

Wash and cube the fruits, and place in a salad bowl. Mix lemon juice, sugar substitute, and rum. Pour the obtained syrup over fruits and toss to coat. Move the fruit salad into serving cups, and refrigerate for ½ hour before serving.

Serves: 2

Sunshine Salad

(3 ounce) package, sugar-free lemon flavored gelatin
1 cup boiling water
1 cup cold water
1 cup green apple, chopped
1 cup grapefruit, chopped
1 teaspoon white wine vinegar
½ teaspoon cinnamon powder
¼ cup chopped walnuts (optional)

Dissolve gelatin in boiling water. Add cold water, vinegar, and cinnamon. Chill until partially set. Fold in apple, grapefruit and walnuts. Pour into molding cups. Chill until firm.

Serves: 2

Cheese Pudding

½ pound part-skim ricotta cheese
½ cup Splenda sugar substitute
1 cup egg whites
1 cup egg substitute
½ teaspoon cinnamon powder
1 tablespoon lemon zest
1 teaspoon rum
2 tablespoons wheat germs

Preheat oven at 350 degrees. Mix cheese and sugar substitute with electric mixer. Add egg whites and continue to mix; add egg substitute, lemon, rum, cinnamon, beating well after each addition. Spray a 4-cup ring mold with nonstick cooking spray; lightly sprinkle with wheat germs. Place cheese mixture into the mold. Bake in shallow pan of hot water for 1 hour or until knife inserted in center comes out clean.

Serves: 4

Stuffed Baked Apples

4 apples, cored and cut in half
1 tablespoon part-skim ricotta cheese
1 teaspoon rum
½ teaspoon cinnamon powder
1 tablespoon egg whites
1 tablespoon walnuts chopped

Scoop out small cave in center of each apple half. Mix well apple pulp with ricotta cheese, rum, cinnamon, and egg whites. Fill apple halves with mixture. Top with walnuts. Bake at 350 degrees until apples are tender.

Serves: 4

Baked Apples

6 large apples
4 teaspoons ground cinnamon
1 teaspoon vanilla extract
1½ cup water

Core and wash apples. Place apples in ungreased baking dish. Place ¼ teaspoon ground cinnamon in center of each apple. Sprinkle apples generously with cinnamon. Pour water into baking dish. Add vanilla extract into water. Bake at 375 degrees for 40 minutes or until tender. Cool and spoon syrup over the apples.

Serves: 6

Apple Ricotta Pie

2 large apples
4 tablespoons part-skim ricotta cheese
2 tablespoons egg whites
2 tablespoons egg substitute
1 teaspoon vanilla extract
2 teaspoons ground cinnamon
2 tablespoons walnuts, minced
1 tablespoon wheat germs

Peel apples and cut in thin slices. Arrange slices to cover the entire bottom of a baking dish. Sprinkle with cinnamon and bake at 375 degrees until fork tender. Remove from oven. Beat egg whites until stiff. Mix ricotta cheese, egg substitute, wheat germ, and vanilla extract until smooth. Incorporate egg whites into cheese mixture. Sprinkle walnuts over baked apples. Put cheese mixture on top to make even layer. Return to oven and bake for additional 15 minutes. Cool and slice.

Serves: 4

Fudge Delight

¼ pound dark chocolate
2 tablespoons unsalted butter
2 tablespoons egg whites, well beaten
1 tablespoon coffee cream
½ teaspoon vanilla
½ teaspoon rum
2 tablespoons walnuts, chopped
1 cup Splenda sugar substitute

Melt chocolate and butter in double boiler. Mix egg whites with sugar substitute. Add coffee cream, vanilla, and rum. Combine with melted chocolate. Stir until well blended. Pack in a sprayed with non stick cooking spray, 8-inch pan. Sprinkle on top with walnuts. Cut into desired squares.

Serves: 10

Stuffed Crepes

This is my mom recipe. Good thing about it is that you can make it a dessert or a meal. For a dessert you can use any sugar-free jam, or sweet cheese. You can use fresh fruits and sugar-free whip cream, or you can use sugar-free ice cream. As a dessert serve on a warm plate, sprinkle some Splenda on top and around it, add two strawberries and fresh mint leaves and you can serve restaurant like dessert.

Crepes:
1½ cups soy flour/ Spelt flour
½ teaspoon baking powder
½ teaspoon salt
2 cups 2%fat milk or carbonated water if you have
1 cup egg substitute

Filling:
2 cups small curd 2%fat cottage cheese
1 cup fat-free fetta cheese, crumbled
1 cup egg substitute

2 cups low-fat sour cream.
1 tablespoon fresh parsley, chopped

Mix well all ingredients, less sour cream, until well blend.

For crepes:
Mix flour, baking powder, and salt in a medium bowl. Stir in egg substitute and milk. Beat with hand beater or electric one if you have, until smooth. Spray a skillet with nonstick cooking spray and heat over medium heat. For each crepe, pour ¼ cup batter into skillet; immediately rotate skillet until thin film covers bottom. Cook until light brown. Run wide spatula around the edges to loosen; flip over and cook other side until light brown. Stalk crepes on a plate until all crepes are cooked. Spread cheese mixture evenly on each crepe (approx.1 tablespoon); fold in the sides and roll it up like a burrito. Place stuffed crepes seam down in a baking pan. Mix sour cream until smooth. Pour over crepes and bake in oven at 375 degrees for 20 minutes or until sour cream bubbles.
Serve warm.

Serves: 4

Romanian Style Cream Brûlée

8 tablespoons egg whites
8 tablespoons egg substitute
9 tablespoons Splenda sugar substitute
3 tablespoons sugar
1 teaspoon vanilla
1 teaspoon lemon zest
2 tablespoon rum
4½ cups 2% milk

Heat 3 tablespoons sugar in 2 quarts sauce pan over low heat, stirring constantly, until sugar is melted and golden brown. Pull away form heat. Carefully move sauce pan from side to side and around to coat evenly the entire sauce pan with melted sugar. Let it cool, allowing syrup to harden. Meanwhile, beat egg whites with electric mixer until stiffen. Add one tablespoon at time of the sugar substitute, continuing to beat. Add egg substitute, one tablespoon at the time. Continue to beat. Gradually stir in milk. Add vanilla and lemon zest. Add mixture to sugar coated sauce pan. Place pan in a larger pan filled with water within 1-inch from top. Preheat oven at 350 degrees. Bake for 45 minutes to one hour, or until a knife inserted in middle comes out clean. Set aside, and pour rum evenly around cream. Refrigerate 2 hours before serving.

Serves: 8

Sugar Free Marble Pound Cake

1 ½ cup egg whites
1 ½ egg substitute
9 tablespoons Splenda sugar substitute
8 tablespoons whole wheat flour
8 tablespoons extra-virgin olive oil cold press
1 teaspoon vanilla extract
1 teaspoon lemon zest
1 teaspoon cinnamon
2 tablespoons cacao powder

Beat egg whites with electric mixer until stiff. Gradually, add sugar substitute one tablespoon at the time, continuing to beat. Add gradually egg substitute, beating until combine. Add vanilla extract, lemon zest, and cinnamon. Add whole wheat flour, one tablespoon at the time continuing to beat until combined. Add olive oil, one tablespoon at the time, beating until well incorporated. Preheat oven to 350 degrees. Spray a 9x13x2 baking pan with nonstick cooking spray. Pour mixture into prepared baking pan, reserving 1/3 of it. Add cacao to the reserved mixture and mix well until combined. Spread cacao mixture on top of the mixture in the pan, making your own design. Bake for 45 minutes or until a toothpick inserted in center comes out clean. Cool on wire rack. Cut in squares or any desired shape.

Serves: 8

Chocolate Cake Delight

3 cups whole wheat flour
2 cups Splenda sugar substitute
4 tablespoons cacao powder
2 teaspoons baking powder
½ teaspoon salt
2 cups warm water
2 tablespoons white wine vinegar
1 teaspoon vanilla extract
1 teaspoon rum extract
¾ cup extra-virgin olive oil, cold press

Icing:
1 dark chocolate bar
2 tablespoon 2% fat milk
1 teaspoon rum extract
2 tablespoons ground walnuts

Preheat oven at 350 degrees. In large bowl mix together flour, sugar substitute, salt and cacao powder. In a small cup, mix baking powder and vinegar until the baking powder it is dissolved. Add vinegar mixture to the bowl. Stir in water, vanilla extract, rum extract and oil. Mix well until combined. Spray a 9x13x2 inch baking pan with nonstick cooking spray. Add mixture to the pan and bake for 30 minutes or until a toothpick inserted in center comes out clean. Let it cool in the pan for about 10 minutes. Meanwhile, melt chocolate in a bowl over a pan with boiling water. Add milk, rum extract and walnut. Mix well to blend. Remove form heat. Frost the cake with icing. Cool completely in pan before cutting and serving.

Serves: 8

Cheese Blintzes

1 cup soy flour
½ teaspoon salt substitute
½ teaspoon baking powder
1 cup 2 % fat milk

¾ cup egg substitute
1 tablespoon Smart balance, melted
2 cup 1% fat cottage cheese
2 tablespoons Splenda sugar substitute
1 teaspoon ground cinnamon
¼ teaspoon nutmeg
½ teaspoon vanilla extract

Sift flour, salt and baking powder together. Beat milk, ½ cup egg substitute and Smart Balance. Slowly add to flour mixture. Mix to form thin batter. Spray a 6 inch skillet with nonstick cooking spray. Put over medium heat. Pour 1/8 cup batter into skillet and cover bottom completely. Cook until top is set and bubbly. Flip onto a paper towel. Make rest of pancakes, spraying skillet as necessary. Mix cottage cheese, sugar substitute, cinnamon, nutmeg, vanilla and remaining of egg substitute. Top each pancake on browned side with 1 tablespoon of filling. Fold over sides, then the ends to make store type package. Set aside with flap side down. Refrigerate. To serve, spray a skillet with nonstick cooking spray, place over medium heat and lightly brown each blintz starting with flap side down. Put 2 blintzes on a desert plate, put 1 teaspoon low-fat sour cream (optional) on top, garnish with mint leaves, and sprinkle with sugar substitute on plate around blintze.

Serves: 4

Hot Chocolate

3 oz unsweetened dark chocolate, cut up
2 tablespoons Splenda, sugar substitute
½ teaspoon ground cinnamon
¼ teaspoon cardamon
4 cups 2% fat milk
¼ teaspoon vanilla extract
Sugar-free whipped cream

In a blender or food processor combine chocolate, sugar substitute, cinnamon and cardamon. Process or blend until mixture is finely ground. In a large sauce pan, combine chocolate mixture and milk. Cook and stir over low heat until chocolate melts, about 10 minutes. Remove from heat, add vanilla extract and beat with a rotary beater until frothy. Top with 1 teaspoon of whipped cream before serving.

Serves: 4

Truffles

1 package 12-oz. unsweetened chocolate
1 cup Splenda sugar substitute
1 cup heavy cream
2 tablespoons fat-free, sugar-free, whip cream
1 teaspoon rum extract
¼ cup ground almonds

To coat:
Cacao powder mixed with 1 teaspoon cinnamon
Ground walnuts mixed with 1 tablespoon sugar substitute

Melt chocolate in a double boiler. Remove from heat. Stir in sugar substitute, heavy cream and rum extract. Fold in whip cream and almonds. Refrigerate for 30 minutes or until thick enough to hold a shape. Line a cookie sheet with parchment paper. Drop mixture by teaspoonfuls onto cookie sheet, and shape into balls. Refrigerate for 10 minutes. Coat truffles with cacao powder or ground walnuts, by taking one ball at the time and roll it onto the coating. Return coated truffles to the cookie sheet. You can store truffles in airtight container.

Serves: 10

Chocolate Covered Truffles

Truffles
1 package 12-oz. unsweetened chocolate
1 cup Splenda sugar substitute
¼ cup heavy cream
4 tablespoons sugar-free, fat-free whip cream
1 teaspoon raspberries extract

To coat:
6-oz. unsweetened chocolate
½ cup sugar substitute
1 tablespoon unsalted butter

Melt chocolate in a double boiler. Remove from heat. Stir in sugar substitute, heavy cream and raspberries extract. Fold in whip cream. Refrigerate for 30 minutes or until thick enough to hold a shape. Line a cookie sheet with parchment paper. Drop mixture by teaspoonfuls onto the cookie sheet. Shape into balls. Freeze for 20 minutes. Melt 6 oz. chocolate in a double boiler, stirring constantly. Remove from heat. Stir in sugar substitute and butter. Dip truffles one at the time into chocolate mixture. Return truffles to parchment paper.
Refrigerate for 10 minutes or until coating is set.

Serves: 1

Sugar Free Chocolate Cups Pudding

Chocolate cups:
½ cup unsweetened chocolate chips
1 tablespoon Splenda sugar substitute
1 teaspoon shortening

In a microwave, melt chips and shortening, and stir until smooth. Stir in sugar substitute. With a small pastry brush, spread chocolate mixture on the inside of 1-inch foil or paper candy cups. Place on a baking sheet and refrigerate for 45 minutes or until firm. Just before serving remove foil or paper cups. Using 1 sugar-free, fat-free, vanilla instant, store bought pudding box, make the pudding following the directions on the box. Use 2% fat milk. To serve, fill each chocolate cup with vanilla pudding. Top each cup with fresh raspberries.

Serves: 4

———— Appendix 1 ————

LabCorp Laboratory Corporation of America
LabCorp Dublin
6370 Wilcox Road, Dublin, OH 43016-1296   Phone:

SPECIMEN	TYPE	PRIMARY LAB	REPORT STATUS		
	S	CB	COMPLETE	Page #:	1

ADDITIONAL INFORMATION	SS#:

FASTING: N
PHONE: DOB:

PATIENT NAME	SEX	AGE(YR./MOS.)
MARIAN	M	49 / 5

PT. ADD.:

DATE OF SPECIMEN	TIME	DATE RECEIVED	DATE REPORTED	TIME	
7/20/2007	12:05	7/20/2007	7/21/2007	12:13	109

CLINICAL INFORMATION
CD-

PHYSICIAN ID.	PATIENT ID.
DEFOREST J	

ACCOUNT: John R. DeForest, D.O.

715 Dixie Highway
Beecher   IL   60401-0000
ACCOUNT NUMBER:

TEST	RESULT		LIMITS	LAB
Comp. Metabolic Panel (14)				
> Glucose, Serum	268 H	mg/dL	65 – 99	CB
Please Note: Specimen is lipemic.				
BUN	20	mg/dL	5 – 26	CB
Creatinine, Serum	1.0	mg/dL	0.5 – 1.5	CB
BUN/Creatinine Ratio	20		8 – 27	
> Sodium, Serum	134 L	mmol/L	135 – 148	CB
Potassium, Serum	4.8	mmol/L	3.5 – 5.5	CB
Chloride, Serum	98	mmol/L	96 – 109	CB
Carbon Dioxide, Total	26	mmol/L	20 – 32	CB
Calcium, Serum	9.8	mg/dL	8.5 – 10.6	CB
Protein, Total, Serum	6.9	g/dL	6.0 – 8.5	CB
Albumin, Serum	4.2	g/dL	3.5 – 5.5	CB
Globulin, Total	2.7	g/dL	1.5 – 4.5	
A/G Ratio	1.6		1.1 – 2.5	
Bilirubin, Total	0.5	mg/dL	0.1 – 1.2	CB
Alkaline Phosphatase, Serum	73	IU/L	25 – 150	CB
AST (SGOT)	16	IU/L	0 – 40	CB
ALT (SGPT)	21	IU/L	0 – 40	CB
Lipid Panel With LDL/HDL Ratio				
> Cholesterol, Total	348 H	mg/dL	100 – 199	CB
> Triglycerides	2200 H	mg/dL	0 – 149	CB
Results confirmed on				
dilution.				
> HDL Cholesterol	39 L	mg/dL	40 – 59	CB
VLDL Cholesterol Cal		mg/dL	5 – 40	
The calculation for the VLDL cholesterol is not valid when				
triglyceride level is >400 mg/dL.				
LDL Cholesterol Calc		mg/dL	0 – 99	
Triglyceride result indicated is too high for an accurate LDL				
cholesterol estimation.				
LDL/HDL Ratio		ratio units	0.0 – 3.6	
Unable to calculate result since non-numeric result obtained for				
component test.				

	LDL/HDL	
	Men	Women
1/2 Avg.Risk	1.0	1.5
Avg.Risk	3.6	3.2
2X Avg.Risk	6.3	5.0
3X Avg.Risk	8.0	6.1

Pat Name:	MARIAN	Pat ID:	Spec #:	Seq #: 109

Results are Flagged in Accordance with Age Dependent Reference Ranges
Continued on Next Page

Appendix 2

FOODS TO YOUR ADVANTAGE

To Lower Cholesterol Level

ALMONDS: are rich on monounsaturated fat; can lower LDL cholesterol (low density lipoprotein) commonly known as the bad cholesterol. They are also a high source of vitamin E, an anti-inflammatory nutrient recommended ½ cup per day.

APPLES: are rich in pectin, the fiber that binds to cholesterol, and keeps it from getting into the blood. Pectin is a soluble fiber which slows down the absorption of nutrients into the bloodstream, helping to keep blood sugar under control.

ARTICHOKES: contains luteolin which acts as an antioxidant, and prevents the oxidation of LDL cholesterol. It is also a rich source of cynarin, which helps reducing cholesterol production.

AVOCADO: is a rich source of potassium, a mineral vital for lowering blood pressure. It also contains Beta-silosterol, which can inhibit the absorption of cholesterol from intestines, so it is less into the blood stream. It is a rich source of unsaturated fat which helps lower LDL (bad cholesterol), while maintaining the HDL (good cholesterol).

BARLEY: contains beta-glucan, a type of fiber that lowers cholesterol by trapping some fat and cholesterol from foods and eliminates them before they can be absorbed.

BEANS: are high in both, the soluble fiber which is a cholesterol controller and insoluble fiber which is a colon cancer fighter.

BLACKBERRIES: one of the chemicals blackberries contain helps lower cholesterol levels especially LDL cholesterol.

CANOLA OIL: is the only cooking oil rich in heart-healthy alphalinolenic acid, known to lower LDL cholesterol and triglycerides.

CAYENNE, RED PEPPER: contain capsaicin, an antioxidant which helps to lower LDL cholesterol, and reduce the stickiness of blood platelets, so they don't clot.

CACAO: is rich in flavonoids, which has been shown to prevent oxidation of LDL cholesterol; when LDL is oxidized, it clings to arteries and increases the risk of heart disease and stroke. Also, helps to raise levels of HDL cholesterol.

CRANBERRIES: unsweetened cranberry juice could raise HDL (good cholesterol).

GARLIC: contain chemical components known to lower cholesterol.

GINGER: one of the chemicals in ginger called "zingerone" keeps LDL cholesterol from being oxidized.

GINSENG: it is known to raise HDL (good cholesterol).

GRAPEFRUIT: is loaded with pectin; a type of fiber that essentially attaches to cholesterol molecules in intestine and drags them out of body in stools. So that cholesterol never gets into blood stream.

MUSHROOMS: shiitake mushrooms can lower very low density (VLDL) cholesterol.

NUTS: like walnuts and almonds can lower cholesterol.

OLIVE OIL: is a rich source of unsaturated fat, which can lower LDL cholesterol.

ONION: contain quercetin, which can help prevent free radicals from damaging LDL cholesterol; process that makes it more likely to gunk up the arteries

ORANGES: are rich in pectin (white pith under the orange skin) the type of fiber that lowers cholesterol.

PARSLEY: contain terpenoids, a compound that can reduce level of LDL.

PRUNES: contain neochlorogenic acid, an antioxidant which prevents the oxidation of LDL cholesterol; a process that leads to clogged arteries.

TOFU: it is a processed form of soy; contains antioxidants which may lower cholesterol.

To Lower Blood Pressure

APPLES: are excellent potassium sources; potassium prevents thickening of the artery walls and works in conjunction with sodium to regulate body's fluid levels. Excess fluid in arteries can elevate blood pressure.

AVOCADO: it is a good source of potassium, which is vital for lowering blood pressure.

BEETS: are rich sources of betacyanin, which may help cells take in more oxygen.

One cup of fresh beets delivers 1/3 of daily requirement for folate-B vitamin.

BLUEBERRIES: are rich sources of bioflavonoids, antioxidants which help to strengthen cardiovascular system and prevent molecular damage. They are also, rich in fiber, which has a role in lowering systolic blood pressure.

BOK CHOY: is good source of calcium; it is known that calcium and magnesium help reduce the tension in artery walls and relax the muscles that control blood vessels.

BROCCOLI: has a high content in magnesium and potassium, which helps controlling blood pressure.

CANTALOUPE: contains potassium which reduces the risk of high blood pressure. Also it is rich source of Beta-carotene which is a plant chemical that's converted to vitamin A in the body. Beta-carotene can also be found sweet potatoes, and winter squash.

CARDAMON: it is a spice that may help stimulate antioxidant enzymes in the body. Blocking oxidation helps prevent cholesterol from sticking to the walls of arteries, thus prevent heart disease.

CAULIFLOWER: it is a rich source of biotin-B vitamin which helps the body to make and use amino acids, the building block of proteins. It is also rich in vitamin C, which protects the heart by consuming free radicals, compounds, known to play an important role in developing heart disease. Also contains folate-B vitamin that has a role on lowering levels of amino acids.

CELERY: is rich in 3-n-butyl phthalite which acts as a diuretic and vasodilator and helps relax the muscles lining the blood vessels.

COENZYME Q 10 (CoQ10): found in salmon and tuna, it is a powerful antioxidant that appears to bring oxygen to the heart and even help curb the damage caused by lack of oxygen. Also, makes arteries less vulnerable to constriction.

GARLIC: row, inhabits blood clots that can cause heart attack, and reduces blood pressure. Garlic contains allicin, known to have a blood thinning effect.

GINGER: inhibits clotting of platelets in blood which reduces the risk of a heart attack.

GRAPEFRUIT: contains lycopene, a carotenoid, a plant pigment that is believed to have powerful antioxidant properties, important key to a healthy heart.

HORSERADISH: is rich in vitamin C, essential nutrient for preventing heart disease, because it helps stop harmful free radicals from damaging lining of arteries and encouraging the accumulation of cholesterol deposits.

MEAT: only lean cuts of red meat contain carnitine which is an amino acid that may help strengthen the heart muscle.

MUSHROOMS: may help prevent circulatory disease. Shiitake and Maitake mushrooms appear to lower blood pressure.

NUTS: are rich in selenium, a mineral that appears to play a role in keeping arteries clear.

OMEGA -3: found in salmon, represents a key role in preventing heart disease, and may help lower blood pressure.

ONIONS: are rich in quercetin which seems to be more powerful then vitamin E at blocking the harmful effects of free radicals. They also contain adenosine and paraffinic polysulfide, a chemical compounds which keep blood platelets from clumping together to form clots. They are a rich source of selenium, a mineral, a powerful antioxidant that helps keeping arteries clear and known to lower triglycerides level.

SPINACH: it is packed with coenzyme Q10, which appears to help bring oxygen to the heart. It is rich in vitamin E, an antioxidant which prevents oxidative damage in cells. It is also a good source of magnesium, a mineral that relaxes smooth muscles, including those that encircle blood vessels.

STRAWBERRIES: are rich sources of fiber; the fiber in fruit apparently works even better than the fiber in vegetables and grains to lower systolic blood pressure. They are also rich in antioxidants.

TOMATOES: are rich in lycopene, a carotenoid which has powerful antioxidant properties, and helps prevent harmful molecules in the body from damaging healthy cells in the arteries.

TURMERIC: it is a spice, which is known to inhibit arterial inflammation.

Other

BEANS: are rich in insoluble fiber, which is a colon cancer fighter.

EVENING PRIMROSE: it is oil that seems to balance hormones, support the immune system, and reduce inflammation.

GINGER: may help to raise both, the body temperature and the metabolism.

GINSENG: can lower blood sugar level, by slowing down digestion, and decreasing the rate at which carbohydrates are absorbed into blood stream.

LINOLEIC ACID: in supplement form, appears to decrease blood sugar level.

PSYLLIUM: the seeds are loaded with fiber, and it is believed that may lower insulin resistance.

TOMATOES: are rich in lycopene, which may lower the risk of prostate cancer.

VINEGAR: the acid in vinegar slows the conversion of carbohydrates to blood sugar.

BARLEY: it is grain that has no gluten content, which makes it good for diabetics.

Appendix 3

GRANDMA'S KITCHEN TIPS

Those kitchen tips have been passed on to me from generation to generation. My mother had them written down in her always present in the kitchen note book. I found them very helpful, and that is way I decided to share them with you.

EGG WHITES:

To keep fresh egg whites longer, place them in an airtight container, add one tablespoon cold water on top and refrigerate.

Will stiffen faster if you add to it dash salt or dash sugar.

If you add one tablespoon of cold water to the egg whites, when you beat them, for the same quantity of egg whites you will obtain a bigger quantity of stiffen egg whites.

BANANAS

To stop bananas from changing the color, sprinkle with lemon juice.

CHEESE

You can shred any kind of cheese without shattering, if you keep it in the freezer for 30 minutes before.

The best, and easy way to cut any type of frail cheese, is to run the knife through hot water before.

If you like a kind of cheese but you can not eat it because is to salty, you can unsalted the cheese if you wrap the cheese in white paper and keep it in cold water for one hour.

If you have an old piece of cheese, that has been sitting in refrigerator for a while and it got hard, wrap it in towel soaked in dry white wine for one hour. It will become soft again.

BROCCOLI
Choose only ones who have an intense green color, without any yellow spots. Before cooking, separate broccoli in flowerets and keep them in cold water with one tablespoon of vinegar, then rinse in cold water.

BASIL
Basil is great in any vegetable salads, due to its unique taste. Make your own basil oil salad dressing. Here it is how: take fresh basil, rinse and chop. Put it in a jar. Add extra virgin olive oil over. Keep it in refrigerator or in a dark, cold and dry place. It is ready to use after 2 hours.

CALAMARI
Calamari will be softer and delicious, if you soak it in mineral water for twenty minutes before cooking.

MEAT
Fresh meat does not bleed. Meat that was frozen before bleeds a lot when cut. To know if meat is fresh, press down with your finger; if meat regains its shape that means that is fresh.

Lean pork chops will be juice and soft, if you keep them in a mixture of cold water and vinegar for 5 minutes, before cooking. The mixture should be one part of vinegar to two parts of water.

Pork meat will be tendered, if you keep it in yogurt for half on hour, before cooking.

Beef will be tendered and juice if you keep it for two hours in a mixture of olive oil and vinegar, before cooking.

Chicken meat becomes savory if you keep it for one hour in cold milk.

Grilled chicken it is delicious if you marinated before in yogurt and your favorite spices.

POTATOES

Baked potatoes will be ready in 15 minutes if you boil them for 5 minutes, before baking.

Boiled potatoes will peel a lot easier if you rinse them immediately after boiling in cold water.

Always salt fried potatoes at the end to have them crisp.

STRAWBERRIES

Never rinse strawberries after you take the steam out, in order to preserve the juices and vitamins. Strawberries will increase their natural aroma if after rinse you add 1 teaspoon of white vinegar.

BEANS

Green beans have to be cooked right away. If you keep them in the refrigerator, for more then two days, they will become toxic and will generate indigestion.

Dry beans will boil faster if you add to the boiling water 1 teaspoon of baking soda.

Green beans, will keep their color if you add to the boiling water 1 teaspoon of baking soda.

NUTS

Dry walnuts could become fresh, if they are kept for 5 to 6 days in jar with water and 1 tablespoon of salt.

OMELET

Omelet becomes softer and fluffy, if you add water to composition instead of milk.

VINEGAR

If a vinegar taste to strong or it is to concentrate, add 1 sliced apple for 24 hours. Apple it gives a great aroma.

EGGS

To be sure that the eggs are fresh, put the egg into a cup of water; if the egg does go to the bottom that means that it is fresh; if the egg floats that means that it is old.

To make the best poached egg: separate egg white and yolk; add to pan first the egg white and when it is set add the yolk on top, and cook for few more minutes.

When you season your eggs, always season the egg white with salt and the yolk with pepper. Salt leaves spots on the yolk.

You can peel easily boiled eggs if you add 1 teaspoon of salt to boiling.

SPAGHETTI

To boil the perfect spaghetti, add to the water PAM spray, this way you will not only stop the foaming, but they will not stick together, or to the pan.

PARSLEY

Before you chop parsley dump it in hot water. This way you can chop it easy and the aroma intensifies.

The aroma of flat parsley it is stronger then of the curly one, and it is best in salads.

SALAD DRESSING

Invigorating salad dressing: 1½ cup low fat sour cream, juice from 1 orange, juice from ½ lemon, salt and black pepper to taste. Mix well and keep refrigerated.

Appendix 4

NUTRITIVE VALUE OF FOODS USED IN THE RECIPES

Milk and Dairy products

Item Name	Serving size	Total fat g	Sat. fat g	Trans fat g	Cholest mg	Sodium mg	Total carb. g	Sugar g	Protein g
The Laughing Cow light cheese	1 wedge	2	1	0	10	260			
Mini Babybel light cheese	1 piece	3	1.5	0	15	160	0	0	6
Kraft low moisture part-skim Mozzarella cheese	1oz	6	3.5	0	15	200	1	0	7
lucerne low-moisture part-skim mozzarella cheese shredded	¼ cup	5	3	0	15	180	1	0	8
Crystal Farms reduced fat Mozzarella cheese shredded	¼ cup	4	2.5	0	10	180	1	0	7
BelGioioso fresh mozzarella	1oz	6	4	0	20	85	0	0	5

Item Name	Serving size	Total fat g	Sat. fat g	Trans fat g	Cholest mg	Sodium mg	Total carb. g	Sugar g	Protein g
lucerne low fat Ricotta cheese	¼ cup	3	2	0	20	160	3	2	7
Lactaid low fat cottage cheese	½ cup	1	0.5	0	10	380	7	3	12
President fat free crumbled Feta cheese	1oz	0	0	0	5	260	1	0	7
President fat free Feta cheese	1oz	0	0	0	5	450	2	1	6
Daisy light sour cream	2tbsp	2.5	2	0	10	25	2	2	2
Daisy non fat sour cream	2tbsp	0	0	0	0	15	1	1	1
Sorrento part-skim Ricotta cheese	¼ cup	4.5	2.5	0	30	75	4	1	5
Unsweetened soy milk	1cup	4	0.5	0	0	85	4	1	

Other

Item name	Serving size	Total Fat g	Sat. fat g	Trans. fat g	Cholest mg	Sodium mg	Total carb. g	Sugar g	Proteins g
Egg Beaters egg whites	3 tbsp	0	0	0	0	75	1	0	5
Egg Beaters 99% real eggs	¼ cup	0	0	0	0	115	1	1	6
Oasis Classic Cuisine zero-fat hummus	2tbsp	0	0	0	0	37	3	0	1

Vegetables

Item Name	Serving size	Calories	Carb. g	Fiber g	Protein g	Fat g
Artichokes, cooked, drained	1cup	84	19	9.1	6	trace
Asparagus	1cup	43	8	2.9	5	0.3
Beans, green snap raw	1cup	44	10	4	2	trace
Beans, yellow, snap, raw	1cup	44	10	4.1	2	trace
Beans, lima, cooked	1cup	216	39	13.2	15	1
Beets, raw	1cup	58	13.4	1.1	2.2	1
Broccoli, raw	1cup	25	5	2.6	3	trace
Brussels sprouts, raw	9 med.	45	14	4.1	4	1
Cabbage, raw	1cup	18	4	1.6	1	trace
Cabbage, red, raw	1cup	19	4	1.4	1	trace
Carrot, raw	1 large	31	7	2.2	1	trace
Cauliflower flowerets, raw	1cup	25	5	2.5	2	trace
Celery, raw	1cup	19	4	2	1	trace
Chives, raw, chopped	1tbsp	1	trace	0.1	trace	trace
Cucumber	1cup	14	3	0.8	1	trace
Eggplant, raw	1/3 med	28	7	2.5	1	trace
Endive, raw	1cup	9	2	1.6	1	trace
Garlic, raw	1clove	4	1	0.1	trace	trace
Hearts of palm, canned	1 piece	9	2	0.8	1	trace
Lettuce, Boston	head 5"	21	4	1.6	2	trace
Lettuce, Romaine	1 cup	8	1	1	1	trace
Mushrooms, raw	1cup	18	3	0.8	2	trace
Okra, cooked, from raw	1 cup	51	12	4	3	trace
Onions raw, chopped	1 cup	61	14	2.9	2	trace
Onions green, raw, chopped	1 cup	32	7	2.6	2	trace
Parsley, raw	10 sprigs	4	1	0.3	trace	trace
Parsnip, cooked	1 cup	126	30	6.2	2	trace
Peas, edible pod, cooked, from raw	1 cup	67	11	6.2	5	trace
Peppers, green, raw	1 cup	40	10	2.7	1	trace
Peppers, red, raw	1 cup	40	10	3	1	trace
Radishes, raw	1 radish	1	trace	0.1	trace	trace
Shallots, raw, chopped	1 tbsp	7	2	0.2	trace	trace
Sauerkraut, canned	1 cup	45	10	5.9	2	trace
Soybeans, green, cooked	1 cup	254	20	7.6	22	12
Spinach, raw, chopped	1 cup	7	1	0.8	1	trace
Squash, summer, raw	1cup	23	5	2.1	1	trace
Squash, winter, baked, cubes	1cup	80	18	5.7	3	trace
Sweet potatoes, baked with skin	1potato	150	35	4.4	3	trace
Sweet potatoes, boiled	1potato	164	38	2.8	3	trace
Tomatillos, raw	1 medium	11	2	0.6	trace	trace

Item Name	Serving size	Calories	Carb. g	Fiber g	Protein g	Fat g
Tomatoes, raw, chopped	1 cup	38	8	2	2	1
Tomatoes, raw, whole	1 medium	26	6	1.4	1	trace
Tomatoes, raw, cherry	1 cherry	4	1	0.2	trace	trace
Tomato juice, canned	1 cup	41	10	1	2	trace
Tomato paste	2tbsp	25	6	2	1	0
Turnips, cooked, cubes	1 cup	33	8	3.1	1	trace

Legumes, Nuts, and Seeds

Item Name	Serving size	Calories	Carb. g	Fiber g	Protein g	Fat g
Almonds, shelled, sliced	¼ cup	180	6	3	8	14
Beans, black, dry, cooked	1 cup	227	41	15	15	1
Beans, kidney, red	1 cup	225	40	13.1	15	1
Beans, lima, large	1 cup	216	39	13.2	15	1
Black eyed peas, dry, cooked	1 cup	200	36	11.2	13	1
Chickpeas, dry, cooked	1 cup	269	45	12.5	15	4
Hummus, commercial	1 tbsp	23	2	0.8	1	1
Lentils, dry, cooked	1 cup	230	40	15.6	18	1

Fruits

Item Name	Serving Size	Calories	Carb. g	Fiber g	Protein g	Fat g
Apple, raw, unpeeled	1 apple	81	21	3.7	trace	trace
Avocados, raw, without skin and seed	1 oz	32	3	1.5	trace	3
Blackberries, raw	1 cup	75	18	7.6	1	1
Blueberries, raw	1 cup	81	20	3.9	1	1
Cantaloupe, raw, without rind	1 wedge	24	6	0.6	1	trace

Item Name	Serving Size	Calories	Carb. g	Fiber g	Protein g	Fat g
Grapefruit, raw, without peel	½ grapefruit	37	9	1.4	1	trace
Lemons, raw, without peel	1 lemon	17	5	1.6	1	trace
Lemon juice, raw	juice of 1 lemon	12	4	0.2	trace	0
Lime juice, raw	juice of 1 lime	10	3	0.2	trace	trace
Oranges, raw, without peel and seeds	1 orange	62	15	3.1	1	trace
Pears, raw, with skin, cored	1 pear	98	25	4	1	1
Raspberries, raw	1 cup	60	14	8.4	1	1
Strawberries, raw, capped	1 strawberry large	5	1	0.4	trace	trace

Meat, Poultry, and Meat products

Item Name	Serving size	Calories	Fat g	Sat. fat g	Trans. fat g	Cholest mg	Sodium mg	Protein g
Ground Beef 80% lean	4 oz	287	23	23	0	80	76	20
Beef, steak, sirloin, broiled	3 oz	166	6	2.4	0	76	72	26
Perdue chicken breast, skinless, boneless	½ chicken breast	140	1.5	0.5	0	90	60	32
Jennie O turkey breast	4 oz	120	1.5	0.5	0	50	75	26
Perdue ground lean turkey	4 oz	130	7	2	0	90	85	21
Canadian bacon	3 slices	60	1.5	0.5	0	30	460	11

Fish and Shellfish

Item Name	Serving size	Calories	Total Fat g	Sat. Fat g	Cholesterol mg	Protein g
Cod, baked or broiled	1 fillet	89	1	0.1	42	21
Crabmeat, canned	1 cup	134	2	0.3	120	28
Roughy, orange, baked or broiled	3 oz	76	1	trace	20	16
Salmon	4 oz	135	1	1	85	23

Item Name	Serving size	Calories	Total Fat g	Sat. Fat g	Cholesterol mg	Protein g
Salmon, smoked	3 oz	99	4	0.8	20	16
Shrimp, peeled and deveined	4 oz	70	0	0	110	16
Shrimp, canned, drained, solids	3 oz	102	2	0.3	147	20
Tuna, baked or broiled	3 oz	118	1	0.3	49	25
Tuna, water pack, solid white	3 oz	109	3	0.7	36	20

Grain Products

Item Name	Serving size	Calories	Total fat g	Sat. Fat g	Sodium mg	Total carb. g	Fiber g	Protein g
All Bran, cereal	½ cup	79	1	0.2	342	23	9.7	4
Arrowhead Mills organic barley flour	¼ cup	95	1	0	0	19	4	5
Bob's Red Mill- 100% whole grain, flaxseed	3 tbsp	160	11	1	10	11	9	6
Bran, wheat	¼ cup	30	0.5	0	0	10	6	2
Buena Vida - whole wheat tortillas	1 tortilla	70	4	1	250	7	3	4
Ceresota 100% whole wheat flour	¼ cup	100	0.5	0	0	21	3	4
Hodgson Mill whole grain stone ground flour	¼ cup	100	1	0	0	22	3	2
Hodgson Mill whole grain, spelt flour	¼ cup	85	1	0	0	21	5	5
Hodgson Mill oat bran, hot cereal	¼ cup	120	3	1	0	23	6	6

Item Name	Serving size	Calories	Total fat g	Sat. Fat g	Sodium mg	Total carb. g	Fiber g	Protein g
Healthy Life" 100% whole grain rye bread	2 slices	80	1	0.5	280	19	7	6
Healthy Harvest, 7 grain blend pasta	2 oz	180	2	0	0	40	5	8
La Tortilla Factory- whole wheat low carb/ low fat tortillas	1 tortilla	50	2	0	180	11	8	5
Mary's Gone Crackers- wheat free, gluten free	15 crackers	80	3.5	1	150	20	3	3
Reese wild rice	¼ cup	166	1	0.1	5	35	3	7
Soy flour	1/3 cup	100	6	2	0	10	2	11

Miscellaneous Items

Item Name	Serving size	Calories	Total Fat g	Sat. Fat g	Cholest. mg	Total Carb. g	Fiber g	Protein g
Bacos bacon flavored bites	1 tbsp	30	1.5	0	0	2	0	3
Bakers unsweetened, baking chocolate squares	8 oz	40	7	4.5	0	4	2	2
Cinnamon	1 tsp	6	trace	0	0	2	1.2	trace
Cocoa powder, unsweetened	1tbsp	30	0.5	0	0	3	1	1
Olives, large pitted	4 olives	25	2.5	1	0	1	0	1
Morton salt substitute	¼ tbsp	0	0	0	0	0	0	0

Data are from the U.S. Department of Agriculture Nutrient Database for Standard References, release 13, and from the manufacturers' labels.

Mention of trade names, commercial products, or companies in this book, is solely for the purpose of providing information and does not imply recommendation or endorsement, over others not mentioned.

Appendix 5

LabCorp LabCorp Dublin
6370 Wilcox Road, Dublin, OH 43016-1296

Phone:

SPECIMEN	TYPE	PRIMARY LAB	REPORT STATUS		
	S	CB	COMPLETE	**Page #:**	1

ADDITIONAL INFORMATION   SS#:

FASTING: N
PHONE: DOB:

PATIENT NAME	SEX	AGE(YR./MOS.)
MARIAN	M	49 / 9

PT. ADD.:

DATE OF COLLECTION TIME	DATE RECEIVED	DATE REPORTED	TIME	
9/08/2005 14:19	9/09/2007	9/09/2007	10:20	1226

CLINICAL INFORMATION
CD-

PHYSICIAN ID.	PATIENT ID.
DEFOREST J	

ACCOUNT: John R. DeForest, D.O.

715 Dixie Highway
Beecher   IL   60401-0000
ACCOUNT NUMBER:

TEST	RESULT		LIMITS	LAB
Comp. Metabolic Panel (14)				
> Glucose, Serum	111 H	mg/dL	65 - 99	CB
BUN	25	mg/dL	5 - 26	CB
Creatinine, Serum	1.0	mg/dL	0.5 - 1.5	CB
BUN/Creatinine Ratio	25		8 - 27	
Sodium, Serum	137	mmol/L	135 - 148	CB
Potassium, Serum	4.5	mmol/L	3.5 - 5.5	CB
Chloride, Serum	101	mmol/L	96 - 109	CB
Carbon Dioxide, Total	25	mmol/L	20 - 32	CB
Calcium, Serum	10.0	mg/dL	8.5 - 10.6	CB
Protein, Total, Serum	6.8	g/dL	6.0 - 8.5	CB
Albumin, Serum	4.3	g/dL	3.5 - 5.5	CB
Globulin, Total	2.5	g/dL	1.5 - 4.5	
A/G Ratio	1.7		1.1 - 2.5	
Bilirubin, Total	0.6	mg/dL	0.1 - 1.2	
Alkaline Phosphatase, Serum	51	IU/L	25 - 150	CB
AST (SGOT)	25	IU/L	0 - 40	CB
ALT (SGPT)	30	IU/L	0 - 55	CB
Lipid Panel With LDL/HDL Ratio				
Cholesterol, Total	199	mg/dL	100 - 199	CB
> Triglycerides	600 H	mg/dL	0 - 149	CB
> HDL Cholesterol	30 L	mg/dL	40 - 59	CB
VLDL Cholesterol Cal		mg/dL	5 - 40	

The calculation for the VLDL cholesterol is not valid when
triglyceride level is >400 mg/dL.

| LDL Cholesterol Calc | | mg/dL | 0 - 99 | |

Triglyceride result indicated is too high for an accurate LDL
cholesterol estimation.

| LDL/HDL Ratio | | ratio units | 0.0 - 3.6 | |

Unable to calculate result since non-numeric result obtained for
component test.

```
                                         LDL/HDL
                                    Men    Women
                   1/2 Avg.Risk 1.0    1.5
                       Avg.Risk 3.6    3.2
                   2X Avg.Risk 6.3    5.0
                   3X Avg.Risk 8.0    6.1
```

Very good

LAB: CB LabCorp Dublin   DIRECTOR: Rose Goodwin A MD

Pat Name:	MARIAN	Pat ID:	Spec #:	Seq #: 1226

Results are Flagged in Accordance with Age Dependent Reference Ranges
Continued on Next Page

258

Appendix 6

Meal Plan and Sugar Level Counts

Meal plan

Day 1: Monday
Sugar level: 129
Breakfast: 2 Vegetables Quiche
Sugar level: 148
Snack: Low-fat cottage cheese and red bell pepper
Sugar level: 129
Lunch: ½ boneless, skinless grilled chicken breast; roasted vegetables; tomato salad
Dessert: Sugar-free gelatin
Sugar level: 150
Snack: 2 wedges Light Laughing Cow cheese; cherry tomatoes
Sugar level: 130
Dinner: Chef's Salad
Dessert: Sugar-free gelatin

Day 2: Tuesday
Sugar level: 138
Breakfast: 1 cup low-fat yogurt
Sugar level: 108
Snack: 4 slices part-skim mozzarella cheese; 4 Flaxseed crackers
Sugar level: 131

Lunch: 1 cup coked whole wheat spaghetti with Piquant Sauce; tossed greens salad with Vinaigrette Sauce
Dessert: Sugar-free gelatin
Sugar level: 166
Snack: Fat-free Hummus and fresh celery
Sugar level: 145
Dinner: Chicken Salad

Day 3: Wednesday
Sugar level: 139
Breakfast: Eggs Benedict
Sugar level: 149
Snack: 2 wedges Light Laughing Cow cheese; 4 Flaxseed crackers
Sugar level: 135
Lunch: Boiled cod; tossed greens salad with vinaigrette sauce
Dessert: Sugar-free gelatin
Sugar level: 132
Snack: Low-fat cottage cheese and red bell pepper
Sugar level: 130
Dinner: Greek Salad

Day 4: Thursday
Sugar level: 120
Breakfast: 1 cup low-fat low-sugar yogurt; ½ cup Fiber One all bran cereal
Sugar level: 124
Snack: Low-fat cottage cheese and fresh radishes
Sugar level: 130
Lunch: ½ grilled chicken breast; 1 cup white rice pilaf; tossed greens salad with vinaigrette sauce
Dessert: ½ cup fresh strawberries
Sugar level: 194
Snack: 1 stick part-skim mozzarella cheese
Sugar level: 149
Dinner: Chicken Salad
Dessert: Sugar-free gelatin

Day 5: Friday
Sugar level: 113

Breakfast: 1 cup low-fat low-sugar yogurt; ½ cup steel cut oatmeal cereal
Sugar level: 137
Snack: 1 wedge Light Laughing Cow cheese; 4 Flaxseed crackers
Sugar level: 112
Lunch: Grilled Mahi Mahi; 1 cup mashed potatoes; Tomato Salad I
Dessert: Sugar-free gelatin
Sugar level: 198
Snack: Fat-free cottage cheese and green bell pepper
Sugar level: 148
Dinner: Chicken Salad
Dessert: Sugar-free gelatin

Day 6: Saturday
Sugar level: 112
Breakfast: 2servings vegetable quiche
Sugar level: 128
Snack: Fat-free cottage cheese and red bell pepper
Sugar level: 120
Lunch: Meat Loaf; Zucchini Patties; endive salad with vinaigrette sauce
Dessert: Sugar-free gelatin
Sugar level: 120
Snack: 1stick part-skim mozzarella cheese
Sugar level: 112
Dinner: Italian Salad

Day 7: Sunday
Sugar level: 111
Breakfast: Mushroom Omelet
Sugar level: 112
Snack: Cottage cheese Delight and grape tomatoes
Sugar level: 110
Lunch: Tuna Burgers
Dessert: Sugar-free gelatin
Sugar level: 114
Snack: Romanian style Eggplant Dip with fresh celery
Sugar level: 120
Dinner: Gaspacho; ½skinless, boneless grilled chicken breast; Mr. Benny's mozzarella salad

Day 8: Monday
Sugar level: 122
Breakfast: 2 Bran Muffins
Sugar level: 111
Snack: 4 part-skim mozzarella cheese slices and red bell pepper
Sugar level: 95
Lunch: Broccoli Soup; Cauliflower Salad
Dessert: Sugar-free gelatin
Sugar level: 86
Snack: Fat-free Hummus and fresh celery
Sugar level: 98
Dinner: Stuffed Eggplant; Cabbage Salad

Day9: Tuesday
Sugar level: 94
Breakfast: 1 cup low-fat low-sugar yogurt; ½cup Bran cereal
Sugar level: 108
Snack: Fat-free cottage cheese and grape tomatoes
Sugar level: 111
Lunch: Greek Eggplant; ½skinless, boneless grilled chicken breast; Tomato Salad II
Sugar level: 118
Snack: 1 wedge Light Laughing Cow cheese; 4 Flaxseed crackers
Sugar level: 111
Dinner: Chef's Salad
Dessert: Sugar-free gelatin

Day 10: Wednesday
Sugar level: 80
Breakfast: Vegetable Omelet; unsweetened bilberry tea
Sugar level: 83
Snack: 1 stick part-skim mozzarella cheese and red bell pepper
Sugar level: 77
Lunch: Salmon Delight; Three Bean Salad
Dessert: Sugar-free gelatin
Sugar level: 83
Snack: Low-fat cottage cheese and grape tomatoes
Sugar level: 81
Dinner: Italian Salad

Day 11: Thursday

Sugar level: 90
Breakfast: 1 cup low-fat low-sugar yogurt; ½ cup Fiber One cereal
Sugar level: 95
Snack: Fat-free Hummus and fresh celery
Sugar level: 93
Lunch: Romanian style Stuffed Peppers
Dessert: Sugar-free gelatin
Sugar level: 103
Snack: Cottage Cheese Delight and green bell peppers
Sugar level: 98
Dinner: Cheese Stuffed Tomatoes

Day 12: Friday

Sugar level: 90
Breakfast: Chicken Frittata
Sugar level: 95
Snack: 1 stick 2% reduced-fat mozzarella cheese
Sugar level: 88
Lunch: Tomato Soup; Oriental Celery
Dessert: Sugar-free gelatin
Sugar level: 85
Snack: Romanian style Eggplant Dip with fresh celery
Sugar level: 83
Dinner: Eggplant Moussaka; Red Cabbage Salad

Day 13: Saturday

Sugar level: 92
Breakfast: 1 Blueberry Muffin; 1 cup unsweetened soy milk
Sugar level: 111
Snack: low-fat cottage cheese and fresh radishes
Sugar level: 98
Lunch: Cod Fish Balls; Pickled Mushrooms Salad
Dessert: ½ fresh apple
Sugar level: 115
Snack: 3 slices part-skim mozzarella cheese and grape tomatoes
Sugar level: 93
Dinner: Tuna Burgers
Dessert: sugar-free gelatin

Day 14: Sunday
Sugar level: 88
Breakfast: 2 servings Vegetable Quiche; 1 cup low-sugar tomato juice
Sugar level: 90
Snack: 1 wedge Light Laughing Cow cheese; 4 Flaxseed crackers
Sugar level: 98
Lunch: ½ chicken breast with Spicy Sauce; Cabbage Salad
Dessert: Sugar-free gelatin
Sugar level: 115
Snack: Romanian style Eggplant Dip with fresh celery
Sugar level: 100
Dinner: Chicken and Tomatillo Stew; tossed green salad with sauce vinaigrette

Day 15: Monday
Sugar level: 90
Breakfast: Cottage Cheese Pancakes
Sugar level: 98
Snack: 1stick part-skim mozzarella cheese
Sugar level: 88
Lunch: Steak and Sweet Potatoes Casserole; Red Cabbage Salad II
Sugar level: 111
Snack: Cottage Cheese Delight and grape tomatoes
Sugar level: 95
Dinner: Italian Salad
Dessert: Sugar-free gelatin

Day 16: Tuesday
Sugar level: 88
Breakfast: Breakfast Parfait
Sugar level: 80
Snack: 3 slices fresh mozzarella cheese and red bell pepper
Sugar level: 77
Lunch: Chicken Salad Stuffed Tomatoes
Dessert: Stuffed Baked Apples
Sugar level: 90
Snack: 1 wedge Light Laughing Cow cheese with fresh celery
Sugar level: 85
Dinner: Grilled salmon; Easy Asparagus; tossed greens salad

Day 17: Wednesday

Sugar level: 87

Breakfast: 2 Cottage Cheese Pancakes

Sugar level: 95

Snack: Romanian style Eggplant Dip with green bell pepper

Sugar level: 90

Lunch: Santa Fe Chicken Salad

Dessert: Sugar-free gelatin

Sugar level: 91

Snack: 1stick part-skim mozzarella cheese; grape tomatoes

Sugar level: 85

Dinner: Baked salmon; Raw Beet Salad

Day 18: Thursday

Sugar level: 95

Breakfast: Egg white Roll Ups

Sugar level: 89

Snack: Cottage Cheese Delight and red bell pepper

Sugar level: 85

Lunch: Mushroom Stuffed Tomatoes

Dessert: Strawberry Salad

Sugar level: 90

Snack: 1stick part-skim mozzarella cheese and red bell pepper

Sugar level: 88

Dinner: ½ skinless, boneless grilled chicken breast; Cauliflower Salad I

Day 19: Friday

Sugar level: 84

Breakfast: Vegetable Omelet; 1 cup fresh grapefruit

Sugar level: 98

Snack: Low-fat cottage cheese and red bell pepper

Sugar level: 88

Lunch: Chicken Stir-Fry; Tomato Salad II

Dessert: Fruit Salad

Sugar level: 98

Snack: 1 wedge Light laughing Cow cheese; 4 Flaxseed crackers

Sugar level: 95

Dinner: Tuna Salad Stuffed Tomatoes

Dessert: Sugar-free gelatin

Day 20: Saturday
>*Sugar level: 88*
>**Breakfast:** Red Bell Pepper Omelet; 1 cup low-sugar tomato juice
>*Sugar level: 80*
>**Snack:** Cottage Cheese Delight and fresh celery
>*Sugar level: 83*
>**Lunch:** Salmon Soufflé; tossed greens salad with sauce vinaigrette
>**Dessert:** ½fresh apple
>*Sugar level: 101*
>**Snack:** 1stick part-skim mozzarella cheese with red bell pepper
>*Sugar level: 95*
>**Dinner:** Tomato Soup; Santa Fe Chicken Salad

Medication Reduced to ½ Dosage Meal Plan and Sugar Levels

Day 1: Monday
>*Sugar level: 117*
>**Breakfast:** Morning Breakfast Parfait
>*Sugar level: 110*
>**Snack:** 3 slices fresh mozzarella cheese and red bell pepper slices
>*Sugar level: 90*
>**Lunch:** Italian Salad
>*Sugar level: 89*
>**Snack:** 1stick part-skim mozzarella cheese and fresh radishes
>*Sugar level: 88*
>**Dinner:** Grilled salmon; steamed asparagus with Blue Cheese Sauce; tossed greens salad
>**Dessert:** Sugar-free gelatin

Day 2: Tuesday
>*Sugar level: 112*
>**Breakfast:** Red Bell pepper Omelet
>*Sugar level: 99*
>**Snack:** 2 wedges Light Laughing Cow cheese and fresh celery
>*Sugar level: 92*
>**Lunch:** Marinated grilled chicken breast; Oven Roasted Vegetables; Cucumber Salad
>**Dessert:** Sugar-free gelatin
>*Sugar level: 111*

Snack: 1 wedge Light Laughing Cow cheeses; ½green bell pepper, sliced
Sugar level: 96
Dinner: Greek Salad
Dessert: Fresh strawberries

Day 3: Wednesday
Sugar level: 98
Breakfast: 1 cup low-fat low-sugar yogurt; ½ cup Bran cereal
Sugar level: 112
Snack: 2 slices fresh mozzarella cheese; 8 black olives
Sugar level: 97
Lunch: Molded chicken Salad
Desert: 1 slice fresh cantaloupe
Sugar level: 111
Snack: 1 stick part-skim mozzarella cheese; ½red bell pepper, sliced
Sugar level: 108
Dinner: Loin beef steak, grilled; ½ cup wild rice pilaf; tossed salad
Dessert: ½fresh apple

Day 4: Thursday
Sugar level: 140
Breakfast: 1 Bran Muffin; 1 cup 2% reduced-fat milk
Sugar level: 126
Snack: 1 wedge Light Laughing Cow cheese and fresh celery
Sugar level: 111
Lunch: Savory Shrimp over romaine lettuce
Dessert: ½ cup fresh blueberries
Sugar level: 99
Snack: 2 tablespoons low-fat cottage cheese and 6 grape tomatoes
Sugar level: 98
Dinner: Crab Salad
Dessert: Sugar-free gelatin

Day 5: Friday
Sugar level: 95
Breakfast: Vegetable Quiche; 1 cup fresh tomato juice
Sugar level: 97
Snack: 2 slices fresh mozzarella cheese; ¼ red bell pepper, sliced
Sugar level: 98

Lunch: Grilled Mahi Mahi; Stir and Fry Vegetables; Tomato Salad I
Dessert: ½ cup fresh strawberries
    Sugar level: 111
Snack: Fat-free Hummus; ½ green bell pepper, sliced
    Sugar level: 99
Dinner: Chicken Salad Stuffed Tomatoes
Dessert: Sugar-free gelatin

Day 6: Saturday
    Sugar level: 95
Breakfast: 1 Blueberry Muffin; 1 cup low-fat low-sugar yogurt
    Sugar level: 110
Snack: ½ cup Cottage Cheese Delight and fresh celery
    Sugar level: 98
Lunch: Marinated grilled chicken breast; Spinach Salad II
Dessert: ½ fresh apple
    Sugar level: 95
Snack: 1 wedge Light Laughing Cow cheese and fresh celery
    Sugar level: 96
Dinner: Tuna Salad Stuffed Tomatoes
Dessert: Sugar-free gelatin

Day 7: Sunday "indulging day"
    Sugar level: 90
Breakfast: Turkey & Swiss open face sandwich, which includes:
    1 slice light rye bread
    1 slice 98% fat-free turkey breast lunch meat
    1 slice low-fat low-sodium Lorraine Swiss cheese
    1 cup bilberry teal with lemon and Splenda sugar substitute
    Sugar level: 95
Snack: Romanian Style Eggplant Dip and fresh celery
    Sugar level: 98
Lunch: Shrimp Chowder; grilled beef loin steak; Oven Roasted Sweet
    Potato Fries; tossed greens salad
Dessert: Low-fat sugar-free ice cream
    Sugar level: 144
Snack: 1 stick 2% reduced-fat mozzarella cheese
    Sugar level: 124(not to bad)
Dinner: Greek Salad

Day 8: Monday

Sugar level: 116(nice rebound)
Breakfast: 1 Bran Muffin; 1 cup low-fat low-sugar yogurt
Snack: 1 wedge Light Laughing Cow cheese and fresh celery
Sugar level: 111
Lunch: Eggplant Moussaka; Red Cabbage Salad II
Dessert: 1 slice fresh cantaloupe
Snack: 1stick part-skim Mozzarella cheese
Sugar level: 99
Dinner: Crab Salad
Dessert: Sugar-free gelatin

Day 9: Tuesday

Sugar level: 89
Breakfast: Eggs Benedict
Snack: Fat-free cottage cheese and ½ red bell pepper, sliced
Sugar level: 91
Lunch: Grilled cod; steamed green beans with Garlic Sauce II
Dessert: ½ cup fresh raspberries
Snack: 3 slices fresh mozzarella cheese and cherry tomatoes
Sugar level: 94
Dinner: Tomato Soup; marinated grilled chicken breast; Spinach Salad
Dessert: Sugar-free gelatin

Day 10: Wednesday

Sugar level: 91
Breakfast: 1 Bran Muffin; 1 cup low-fat low-sugar yogurt
Snack: 1 wedge Light Laughing Cow cheese and fresh celery
Sugar level: 98
Lunch: Salmon Soufflé; tossed greens salad
Dessert: ½ fresh apple
Snack: 1stick part-skim mozzarella cheese
Sugar level: 109
Dinner: Chicken Salad
Dessert: sugar-free gelatin

Day 11: Thursday

Sugar level: 99
Breakfast: Baked Omelet
Snack: Romanian Style Eggplant Dip and fresh celery

Sugar level: 89
Lunch: Cucumber Soup; Romanian Style Stuffed Peppers
Dessert: Sugar-free gelatin
Snack: Low-fat cottage cheese and ½ red bell pepper, sliced
Sugar level: 92
Dinner: Crab Salad
Dessert: ½ cup fresh strawberries

Day 12: Friday

Sugar level: 90
Breakfast: 1 cup All Bran cereal; 1 cup unsweetened soy milk
Snack: low-fat cottage cheese and grape tomatoes
Sugar level: 98
Lunch: Tuna Burgers
Dessert: 1 slice fresh cantaloupe
Snack: 1 wedge Light Laughing Cow cheese; 4 Flaxseed crackers
Sugar level: 106
Dinner: Chef's Salad
Dessert: Sugar-free gelatin

Medication Reduced to ¼ Dosage Meal Plan and Sugar Levels

Day 1: Saturday

Sugar level: 98
Breakfast: Raspberry Parfait
Snack: 1 stick part-skim mozzarella cheese
Sugar level: 97
Lunch: Grilled chicken breast over ½ cup wild rice; Endive Salad
Dessert: ½ fresh pear
Snack: Low-fat cottage cheese and ½ red bell pepper, sliced
Sugar level: 115
Dinner: Grilled salmon; Andra's cauliflower Delight
Dessert: Sugar-free gelatin

Day 2: Sunday

Sugar level: 103
Breakfast: Eggs Benedict; 1 cup low-sugar tomato juice
Snack: 1 wedge Light Laughing Cow cheese; 4 Flaxseed crackers
Sugar level: 99

Lunch: Grilled beef loin steak; Oven sweet Potato Fries; tossed greens salad
Dessert: 1 cup fresh strawberries
Snack: Fat-free Hummus and fresh celery
   Sugar level: 136
Dinner: Ricotta Eggplant Rolls
Dessert: Sugar-free gelatin

Day 3: Monday
   Sugar level: 111
Breakfast: Mushroom Omelet
Snack: 1 stick part-skim mozzarella cheese
   Sugar level: 98
Lunch: Grilled Orange Roughy; Celery and Black Olives, tossed salad
Dessert: 1 slice fresh cantaloupe
Snack: Low-fat cottage cheese and grape tomatoes
   Sugar level: 96
Dinner: Chicken Salad Stuffed Tomatoes
Dessert: Sugar-free gelatin

Day 4: Tuesday
   Sugar level: 99
Breakfast: ½ cup All Bran cereal; low-fat low-sugar yogurt
Snack: 4 slices fresh mozzarella cheese and fresh radishes
   Sugar level: 104
Lunch: Grilled chicken breast; Oven Roasted Vegetables with Sauce Piquant; Red Cabbage salad
Dessert: ½ fresh apple
Snack: 1 wedge Light Laughing Cow cheese; 4 Flaxseed crackers
   Sugar level: 101
Dinner: Tuna meat Balls; Guacamole
Dessert: Sugar-free gelatin

Day 5: Wednesday
   Sugar level: 98
Breakfast: 2 Vegetables Quiche; 1 cup low-sugar tomato juice
Snack: Fat-free Hummus and fresh celery
   Sugar level: 95
Lunch: 2 Chicken Breast Tacos
Dessert: ½ fresh pear
Snack: 1 stick part-skim mozzarella cheese

Sugar level: 113
Dinner: Half grilled chicken breast; Mozzarella cheese Salad
Dessert: Sugar-free gelatin

Day 6: Thursday

Sugar level: 101
Breakfast: Smoked Salmon Quiche; sugar-free bilberry tea with lemon
Snack: ½ cup low-fat cottage cheese and grape tomatoes
Sugar level: 99
Lunch: Grilled chicken breast; Romanian Sweet Potato Salad; tossed salad
Dessert: 1 slice fresh cantaloupe
Snack: 1 wedge Light Laughing Cow cheese; 4 Flaxseed crackers
Sugar level: 116
Dinner: Meat Loaf; Zucchini Patties; tossed salad
Dessert: Sugar-free gelatin

Day 7: Friday

Sugar level: 102
Breakfast: 1 Bran Muffin; sugar-free bilberry tea with lemon
Snack: 1stick part-skim mozzarella cheese
Sugar level: 105
Lunch: Gaspacho; Eggplant Moussaka; tossed salad
Dessert: ½ fresh apple
Snack: 1 Light Mini Babybel cheese and grape tomatoes
Sugar level: 99
Dinner: 2 fish taco
Dessert: Sugar-free gelatin

Day 8: Saturday

Sugar level: 107
Breakfast: low-fat low-sugar yogurt; 1 cup All Bran cereal
Snack: Low-fat cottage cheese; ½ green bell pepper sliced
Sugar level: 103
Lunch: Tomato Soup; Italian Salad
Dessert: ½ cup fresh raspberries
Snack: Fat-free Hummus and fresh celery
Sugar level: 99
Dinner: Grilled salmon; Oriental Celery
Dessert: Sugar-free gelatin

Day 9: Sunday

Sugar level: 97

Breakfast: Turkey Breast Frittata

Snack: Cottage Cheese Delight and cherry tomatoes

Sugar level: 95

Lunch: 2cicken Breast Taco

Dessert: 1Baked Apple

Snack: 1stick mozzarella cheese

Sugar level: 105

Dinner: Greek Salad

Dessert: Sugar-free gelatin

Day 10: Monday

Sugar level: 98

Breakfast: Scrambled eggs (egg substitute)

Snack: Low-fat cottage cheese; ½ red bell pepper sliced

Sugar level: 89

Lunch: 2Romanian Style Stuffed Zucchini; Tomato Salad II

Dessert: 1 slice Apple and Ricotta Pie

Snack: Fat-free Hummus and fresh celery

Sugar level: 98

Dinner: Grilled chicken breast; Creamy Green Beans

Dessert: Sugar-free gelatin

Day 11: Tuesday

Sugar level: 95

Breakfast: 1 Smoked Salmon Quiche; 1 cup low-sugar tomato juice

Snack: Cottage Cheese Delight and fresh celery

Sugar level: 91

Lunch: Dijon Steak; Oven Roasted Sweet Potatoes; tossed salad

Dessert: 1 cup fresh strawberries

Snack: 1stick part-skim mozzarella cheese

Sugar level: 119

Dinner: Italian Salad

Dessert: Sugar-free gelatin

Day 12: Wednesday

Sugar level: 101

Breakfast: 2 Vegetable quiche; 1 cup low-sugar tomato juice

Snack: Fat-free Hummus and fresh celery

Sugar level: 95

Lunch: Lentil Meatball Soup; Spinach Salad
Dessert: 1 slice Romanian Style Crème Brule
Snack: 1stick part-skim mozzarella cheese
  Sugar level: 111
Dinner: Grilled tuna steak; Vegetable stew; tossed salad
Dessert: Sugar-free gelatin

No Medication
Meal Plan and Sugar levels

Day 1: Thursday" The Big Day"
  Sugar level: 101
Breakfast: Raspberry Parfait
Snack: 1stick part-skim mozzarella cheese
  Sugar level: 104
Lunch: Gaspacho; grilled chicken breast; mozzarella salad
Dessert: Sugar-free gelatin
Snack: low-fat cottage cheese; ½ red bell pepper sliced
  Sugar level: 101
Dinner: Chef's Salad
Dessert: ½ fresh apple

Day 2: Friday
  Sugar level: 98
Breakfast: Raspberry Parfait
Snack: 1stick part-skim mozzarella cheese
  Sugar level: 101
Lunch: Romanian Style Baked Salmon; Marinated Mushrooms; tossed salad
Dessert: 1 cup fresh strawberries
Snack: Cottage Cheese Delight and fresh celery
  Sugar level: 99
Dinner: Cheese Stuffed Tomatoes
Dessert: Sugar-free gelatin

Day 3: Saturday
  Sugar level: 95
Breakfast: Low-fat low-sugar yogurt; ½ cup All Bran cereal

Snack: 1stick part-skim mozzarella cheese
Sugar level: 101
Lunch: Grilled salmon; steamed green beans with Sauce piquant; tossed salad
Dessert: ½ fresh apple
Snack: 1 wedge Light Laughing Cow cheese and fresh celery
Sugar level: 103
Dinner: Chef's Salad
Dessert: Sugar-free gelatin

Day 4: Friday
Sugar level: 98
Breakfast: Mushroom Omelet; sugar-free bilberry tea with lemon
Snack: Low-fat cottage cheese and cherry tomatoes
Sugar level: 96
Lunch: Eggplant Moussaka; tossed salad
Dessert: ½ cup fresh blueberries
Snack: 1stick part-skim mozzarella cheese and fresh celery
Sugar level: 95
Dinner: Cauliflower Soup; Meat loaf; tossed salad
Dessert: Sugar-free gelatin

Day 5: Saturday
Sugar level: 91
Breakfast: 2 Vegetable Quiche; 1 cup low-sugar tomato juice
Snack: Romanian Style Eggplant Dip and fresh celery
Sugar level: 95
Lunch: Tomato Soup; Stuffed Eggplant; tossed salad
Dessert: 1 slice fresh cantaloupe, chopped and sprinkled with ground cinnamon
Snack: Low-fat cottage cheese and grape tomatoes
Sugar level: 98
Dinner: Grilled Mahi-Mahi; Pickled Mushrooms Salad
Dessert: Sugar-free gelatin

Day 6: Sunday
Sugar level: 95
Breakfast: 1 Blueberry muffin; sugar-free bilberry tea with lemon
Snack: 1stick part-skim mozzarella cheese and red bell pepper
Sugar level: 100

Lunch: Boiled Cod, tossed salad
Dessert: ½ fresh apple
Snack: Fat-free Hummus and fresh celery
 Sugar level: 98
Dinner: 2 Tuna Burgers
Dessert: Sunshine Salad

Day 7: Monday
 Sugar level: 101
Breakfast: Low-fat low-sugar yogurt; ½ cup All Bran cereal
Snack: Cottage Cheese Delight and green bell pepper
 Sugar level: 99
Lunch: Broccoli Soup; 1 Stuffed Pepper; Tomato Salad
Dessert: ½ cup fresh strawberries
Snack: 1stick part-skim mozzarella cheese and fresh celery
 Sugar level: 92
Dinner: Garlic Eggplant, 2 Tuna Rolls; tossed salad
Dessert: Sugar-free gelatin

Day 8: Tuesday
 Sugar level: 91
Breakfast: Canadian bacon omelet; 1 cup low-sugar tomato juice
Snack: Fat-free Hummus and fresh celery
 Sugar level: 93
Lunch: Roasted salmon; Mashed Spinach; Cucumber Salad
Dessert: ½ cup fresh raspberries
Snack: low-fat cottage cheese and grape tomatoes
 Sugar level: 95
Dinner: Italian Salad
Dessert: Sugar-free gelatin

Day 9: Wednesday
 Sugar level: 92
Breakfast: Turkey Breast Frittata; sugar-free bilberry tea with lemon
Snack: 1stick part-skim mozzarella cheese
 Sugar level: 93
Lunch: Grilled tuna steak with Salsa
Dessert: ½ fresh apple
Snack: Low-fat cottage cheese with grape tomatoes
 Sugar level: 91

Dinner: Chicken Salad Stuffed Tomatoes
Dessert: Sugar-free gelatin

Day 10: Thursday
Sugar level: 90
Breakfast: 2 Vegetable Quiche; low-sugar tomato juice
Snack: 1 wedge Light Laughing Cow cheese and fresh celery
Sugar level: 91
Lunch: Grilled chicken breast; Oven Roasted Vegetables with Pesto
Dessert: ½ cup fresh blueberries
Snack: Fat-free Hummus and fresh celery
Sugar level: 93
Dinner: Tuna Salad Stuffed Tomatoes
Dessert: Sugar-free gelatin

Day 11: Friday
Sugar level: 88
Breakfast: Low-fat low-sugar yogurt; ½ cup Super K cereal
Snack: 1 stick part-skim mozzarella cheese and red bell pepper
Sugar level: 94
Lunch: Grilled salmon; Macedonian Rice; tossed salad
Dessert: Sugar-free gelatin
Snack: Low-fat cottage cheese and grape tomatoes
Sugar level: 108
Dinner: Cheese Stuffed Tomatoes
Dessert: ½ cup fresh Blueberries

Day 12: Saturday
Sugar level: 101
Breakfast: 2 Vegetable Quiche; 1 cup low-sugar tomato juice
Snack: Fat-free Hummus and fresh celery
Sugar level: 93
Lunch: Cabbage Casserole
Dessert*:* ½ fresh apple
Snack: Low-fat cottage cheese; 4 Flaxseed crackers
Sugar level: 101
Dinner: Romanian Style Baked Salmon
Dessert: Sugar-free gelatin

Bibliography

American Dietetic Association. 1997. Diabetes mellitus and exercise. Diabetes Care.20 (suppl.):S51.

American Heart Association. 1996. Statement on exercise: benefits and recommendation for physical activity programs for all Americans. Circulation.94:857-862.

Artal Retal.1996. Exercise: an alternative therapy for gestational diabetes. The Physician and Sports Medicine, 24, 54-66.

Barkman Metal. 1993. The relation between insulin sensitivity and the fatty acid composition of phospholipids in skeletal muscle. New England Journal of Medicine, 328.

Blair, S. N., W. H. Kohl, C.E. Barlow, and L. W. Gibbons. 1991. Physical fitness and all-cause mortality in hypertensive men. Annals of Med. 23:307-312.

Blair, S.N., 1996. Physical inactivity: the public health challenge. Sports Med. Bulletin. 31:3.

Blair, S.N., E. Horton., A.S. Leon, I-M. Lee, B.L. Drinkwater, R. K., Dishman, M. Mackey, and M. L. Kienholz. 1996. Physical activity, nutrition and chronic disease. Med Sci Sports Exerc. 28:335-349.

Blair, S.N., 1993. Evidence for success of exercise in weight loss and control. Ann.Intern.Med119 (7 pt 2):702-706.

Breneman, James C., "Food Allergy," Contemporary Nutrition, 4(March1979), 1-2.

Bjorntorp P.1991. Metabolic implication of body fat distribution. Diabetes Care 14, 1132-1143.

Bjorntorp, P., 1992. Regional fat distribution—implication for type II diabetes. Int J Obes Relat Metab Disord. (16 suppl.)4:S19-27.

Bolourchi, S., C.M. Friedeman, and O. Mickelson.1968. Wheat Flour as source of protein for adult human subjects. Am.J.Clin. Nutr.21:827-835.

Branchtein, L., et al.1997. Waist circumference and waist-to-hip ratio are related to gestational glucose tolerance. Diabetes Care 20, 509-511.

Bray, G.A., 1992. Obesity increases risk for diabetes. Int. J. Obes. Relat. Metab. Disord. (16suppl.)

Bourey, R .E. and S. A. Santora, 1998. Interactions of exercise, coagulation, platelets, and fibrinolysis-a brief review. Med.Sci. Sports. Exerc. 20:439-446.

Burt, V. T., P. Whelton, E. J. Roccela, C. Brown, J. A. Cutler, M. Higgins, M. J. Horans, and D. I. Labarthe. 1995. Prevalence of hypertension in the U.S adult population. Hypertension.25:305-313.

Carl E. Guthe and Margaret Mead, Manual for the study of Food Habits, Bulletin No 111, National Academy of Sciences.

Cartee, G.D. 1994. Influence of age on skeletal muscles glucose transport and glycogen metabolism. Med. Sci Sports Exerc. 26:577-585.

Costill, D.L., E. Coyle, G. Dalsky, W. Evans, W. Fink, and D.Hoopes.1997. Effects of elevated plasma FFA and insulin on muscle glycogen usage during exercise. J. Appl Physiol. 43(4)695-699.

Costill, D.L., A. Bennett, G. Branam, and D Eddy.1973. Glucose ingestion at rest and during prolonged exercise. J Appl Physiol. 34:764-769.

Christiansen MD et al. 1997. Intake of a diet high in trans monounsaturated fatty acids or saturated fatty acids. Diabetes Care 20, 881-887.

Daniel Rosenfield. Protein Quality Testing: Introductory Remarks, Food Tech., Vol.32, No12, 1978, p.51.

Dairy Council Digest 1977. The Role of Dairy Foods in the Diet. Vol.48 No 3.

Das UN 1995. Essential fatty acid metabolism in patients with essential hypertension, diabetes mellitus and coronary heart disease. Prostaglandins Leukotrienes and Essential Fatty Acids52, 387-391.

Devron C.A. et al. (eds.) 1993. Omega 3 Fatty Acids: Metabolism and Biological Effects. Basel: Birkhauser Verlag.

Depres, J.P., C. Bouchard, A. Trembly, R. Savard, and M. Morcotte 1985. Effects of aerobic training on fat distribution in male subjects. Med Sci Sports Exerc.17 (1):113-118.

Durstine, J.L., and W.L. Haskell 1994. Effects of exercise training on plasma lipids and lipoproteins. Exercise and Sports Sciences Reviews.22:477-521.

FAO/WHO.1973. Energy and protein requirements. Report of a joint FAO/ WHO Ad Hoc expert committee. WHO Technical Report Series No.522. Geneva: World Health Organization.

FAO/WHO.1991. Protein Quality Evaluation. Report of a joint FAO/WHO expert consultation. Food and Agricultural Organization Food and Nutrition Paper 51. Rome: FAO.

Flatt J-P. 1995. Use and storage of carbohydrate and fat. American Journal of Clinical Nutrition 61 (suppl.), 952S-959S.

Friedman M.1996. Nutritional value of proteins from different food sources. A review. Journal of Agricultural and Food Chemistry 44, 6-29.

Fabry, P., J.Fodar, Z. Hejl, T. Braun, and K. Zvolankova 1964. The frequency of meals: its relation to overweight, hypercholesterolemia, and decreased glucose-tolerance. Lancet. Sept.19, pp.614-615.

Forbes, G.B. 1973. Another source of error in the metabolic balance method. Nutr. Rev. 31; 297-300.

Fuller, M.F., and P.J. Garlick. 1994. Human amino acid requirements: Can the controversy be resolved? Ann. Rev. Nutr. 14:217-267.

Goodhart, Robert S., and Maurice E. Shils.1980. Modern Nutrition in Health and Disease, Philadelphia: Lea & Febiger, Chapter 7 and 8.

Geliebter et al.1997. Effects of strength or aerobic training on body composition, resting metabolic rate, and peak oxygen consumption in obese dieting subjects. American Journal of Clinical Nutrition 66, 557-563.

Gonzales, Elizabeth Rashe. 1972. Exercise Therapy Rediscovered for Diabetes, But What Does It Do? Journal of the American Medical Association 242:1591.

Hamilton, E.M., and E.N. Whitney .1994. Nutrition Concepts and Controversies, 6th ed. St. Paul: West Publishing Co.

Harris, R.B. 1993. Factors influencing body weight regulation. Dig Dis. 11(3):133-145.

Hill, J.O., and R. Commerford 1996. Physical activity, fat balance and energy balance. Int J Sport Nutr. 6(2):80-92.

Harris, M.B. 1990.Felling fat: motivations, knowledge, and attitudes of overweight women and men. Phych. Reports. 67:1191-1202.

Howard, G. et al.1996. Insulin sensitivity and atherosclerosis. Circulation 93, 1809-1817.

Howlett, T., 1987. Hormonal response to exercise and training: a short review. Clin Endocrin. 26:723-742.

Ivy, J.L.1997. Role of exercise training in the prevention and treatment of insulin resistance and non-insulin-dependent diabetes mellitus. Sports Medicine 24, 321-336.

Jean Mayer, Physiology of Hunger and Satiety; Regulation of Food Intake, in Robert S. Goodhart and Maurice E. Shils (eds.), Modern Nutrition in Health and Disease, Lea & Febiger, Philadelphia, 1973, Chap. 4.

Jepson, M.M., P.C. Bates, and D.J. Millward 1988. The role of insulin and thyroid hormones in the regulation of muscle growth and protein turnover in response to dietary protein. Brit. J. Nutr. 59:397-415.

Luo, J. 1996. Dietary (n-3) polyunsaturated fatty acids improve adipocyte insulin action and glucose metabolism in insulin- resistant rats: relation to membrane fatty acids. Journal of Nutrition 126, 1951-1958.

Landau, B.R.1976. Essential Human Anatomy and Physiology. Glenview, IL: Scott, Foresman.

Leon, A.S., J. Conrod, D.B.Hunninghoke, and R.Serfossi.1979. Effects of a vigorous walking program and body composition, and carbohydrate and lipid metabolism of obese young men. Am J Clin Nutr. 32:1776-1787.

Lehnert, H.R., D.K. Reinstein, B.W. Strowbridge, and R.J. Wurtman.1984a. Neurochemical and behavioral consequences of acute, uncontrollable stress: Effects of dietary tyrosine. Brain Res.303:215-223.

LeRoith, D.1997. Insulin-like growth factors. N. Engl. J. Med. 336:633-640.

Lilliaja, S. et al.1988. Insulin resistance as a precursor of non-insulin dependent diabetes mellitus. Prospective studies of Pima Indians. New England, Journal of Medicine 229, 1988-1992.

Lieberman, H.R., J. Wurtman, and B. Chew.1986b. Changes in mod after carbohydrate consumption among obese individuals. Am. J.Clin. Nutr. 44:772-778.

Marin, P., and P. Bjorntorp.1993. Endocrine-metabolic pattern and adipose tissue distribution. Horm Res. (39 suppl.)3:81-85.

Mayer, J.1968. Overweight: Causes, Cost and Control. Englewood Cliffs, NJ: Prentice- Hall.

Mary, M. Hill. Modification of Food Habits, Food and Nutrition News, Vol. 44, 1972, pp. 1, 4.

Millward, D. J., J. L. Bowtell, P. Pacy, and M.J. Rennie.1994. Physical activity, protein metabolism and protein requirements. Proc. Nutr. Soc. 53(1):223-240.

Mertz, Walter. Effects and Metabolism of Glucose Tolerance Factor. Nutrition Review 33:1929, 1975.

Mikines, K.1988. Effects of physical exercise on sensitivity and responsiveness to insulin in humans. Am J Physiol. 254:E248-E259.

Nair, K.S., D.Halliday, D.E. Matthews, and S.L. Welle.1987. Hyperglucagonemia during insulin deficiency accelerates protein catabolism. Am. J. Physiol. 253:E208-E213.

Owen, O.E., K.J.Smalley, D.A.D'Alessio, M.A. Mozzoli, E.K.Dawson.1998. Protein, fat, and carbohydrate requirements during starvation: anaplerosis and cataplerosis. Am.J.Clin.Nutr. 68:12-34.

Palombo, John D., and George L. Blackburn.1980. Human Protein Requirements. Contemporary Nutrition, 5:1-2.

Pi- Suyner FX 1996. Weight and non-insulin-dependent diabetes mellitus. American Journal of Clinical nutrition 63 (suppl.), 426S-429S.

Pan X-R et al. 1997. Effects of diet and exercise in preventing NIDDM in people with impaired glucose tolerance. Diabetes Care 20, 537-544.

Ross, R.M., and J.S. Jackson.1990. Exercise Concepts, Calculations and Computer applications. Dubuque, IA: Brown & Benchmark.

Sherman, W.M., and A. Albright 1992. Exercise and Type II diabetes. Sports Science Exchange, 4: number 37.

Sarkkinen E. et al. 1996. The effects of monounsaturated-fat enriched diet and polyunsaturated-fat enriched diet on lipid and glucose metabolism in subjects with impaired glucose tolerance. European Journal of Clinical Nutrition 60.

Salmeron J et al.1997. Dietary fiber, glycemic load, and risk of non-insulin dependent diabetes mellitus in men. Diabetes Care 20,545-550.

Shah M., Garg A 1996. High- fat and high-carbohydrate diets and energy balance. Diabetes Care 19, 1142-1152.

Steven D.Garber. Biology A Self-Teaching Guide.1989, John Wiley & Sons, NY.

Tanaka, K., and T. Nakanishi.1996. Obesity as a risk factor for various diseases: necessity of lifestyle changes for healthy aging. Appl Human Sci. 15(4) 139-148.

United States Department of Agriculture and United States Department of Health and Human Services 1995. Nutrition and your Health: Dietary Guidelines for American, 4th ed.

U.S. Department of Health and Human Services. 1993. Second report of the expert panel on detection, evaluation and treatment of high blood cholesterol in adults. Washington, DC: Public Health Service, National Institute of Health. NIH Publication No. 93-3096.

Vranic, M., and D. Wasserman 1990. Exercise, fitness and diabetes. In C. Bouchard, et al. (eds), Exercise, Fitness and Health: A Consensus of Current Knowledge, Champaign, IL: Human Kinetics pp.467-490.

Wardlow, G.M., and P.M. Insel.1996. Perspectives in Nutrition, 3rd ed. St. Louis: Mosby-Year Book Inc.

Wong H. Et al. 1996. Total antioxidant capacity of fruits. Journal of Agriculture and Food Chemistry, 44, 701-705.

Young, C.M., D.L. Frankel, S.S. Scanlan, V. Simko, and L. Lutwok. 1971. Frequency of feeding, weight reduction and nutrient utilization. J Am Diet Assoc. 59:473-480.

Yoshida, A.1983. Specificity of amino acids for the nutritional evaluation of proteins.Pp.163-182 in Proceedings of the International Association of Cereal Chemists Symposium on Amino Acid Composition and Biological Value of Cereal Proteins, R. Lasztity and M. Hidvegi, eds. Budapest: Akademiai Kiado

Index